In a medical emergency, turn immediately to p. 46 in the white (medical) section of this book.

Health Record

Dog's Name: _____

License Number: _____

Where Registered: _____

Veterinarian: _____

             Phone: _____

Date of Birth: _____

Breed: _____

Color: _____

Sex: _____

Date Spayed or Altered: _____

Immunizations against: distemper, leptospirosis, hepatitis, rabies, parainfluenza, and, if appropriate, parvovirus. (Heartworm examinations, medication to prevent infestation, and checks for other types of worms may be included at the time of immunizations.)

Age	Date	Immunizations	Age	Date	Immunizations
___ wks	_____	_____	6 yrs	_____	_____
___ wks	_____	_____	7 yrs	_____	_____
___ wks	_____	_____	8 yrs	_____	_____
1 yr	_____	_____	9 yrs	_____	_____
2 yrs	_____	_____	10 yrs	_____	_____
3 yrs	_____	_____	11 yrs	_____	_____
4 yrs	_____	_____	12 yrs	_____	_____
5 yrs	_____	_____	13 yrs	_____	_____

Treatment of medical problems, excluding worms (To record worming dates, see next page.)

Date   Problem

_____   _____

_____   _____

_____   _____

_____   _____

_____   _____

_____   _____

_____   _____

_____   _____

continued

Treatment of Worms

Type of Worm	Date of Treatment	Type of Treatment
_____	_____	_____
_____	_____	_____
_____	_____	_____
_____	_____	_____
_____	_____	_____
_____	_____	_____
_____	_____	_____
_____	_____	_____
_____	_____	_____

YOUR DOG
AN OWNER'S MANUAL

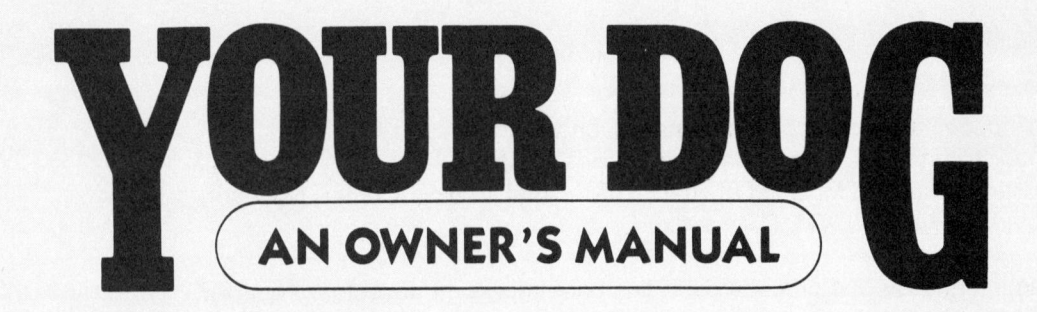

Logical Communications, Inc.

ARCO PUBLISHING, INC.
NEW YORK

This book has been written in consultation with
Brian Kilcommons, Dog Behaviorist, New York, New York
William J. Kay, DVM, Chief of Staff, The Animal Medical Center, New York, New York
Roland G. Oliver, DVM, Brecksville, Ohio

The information and procedures in this book represent accepted practices.
All procedures have been reviewed by the participating consultants.

First Arco Edition, First Printing, 1984

Published by Arco Publishing, Inc.
215 Park Avenue South, New York, N.Y. 10003

Copyright © 1981 by Logical Communications Inc.

All rights reserved. No part of this book may
be reproduced, by any means, without permission
in writing from the publisher, except by a
reviewer who wishes to quote brief excerpts in
connection with a review in a magazine or
newspaper.

Library of Congress Cataloging in Publication Data
Main entry under title:

Your dog.

  1. Dogs—Handbooks, manuals, etc. 2. Dogs—Diseases—
Handbooks, manuals, etc. 3. Dogs—Training—Handbooks,
manuals, etc. I. Logical Communications Inc.
SF427.Y69   1984   636.7   84-9162
ISBN 0-668-06121-9 (Paper Edition)

Printed in the United States of America

10 9 8 7 6 5 4 3 2 1

Foreword

Owning a dog (not being owned by one) is one of the really great experiences of childhood, adulthood, and old age. You are never too young or too old to share your life with a dog and never at a stage where you will not benefit from doing it—*if* you are a person who should own a dog at all.

That *if* is a very, very important word. Read the first section of this manual carefully before you make a commitment to canine companionship. There is nothing wrong with not being a "dog person." There *is* a great deal wrong with owning a dog if you are not.

There is only one way to own a dog, the right way. That means your canine companion is healthy, well-mannered, and well-adjusted to *your* lifestyle. This manual can go a long way toward helping you achieve all three qualities. Without those qualities you are doing something wrong (or failing to do something) and you will not be happy with the long-term results.

Care enough about dog owning to be a good owner. In short, follow the advice—so carefully thought out and constructed for easy reference by Drs. Kay and Oliver and of dog behaviorist and trainer Brian Kilcommons.

—Roger Caras

How to Use
Your Dog: An Owner's Manual

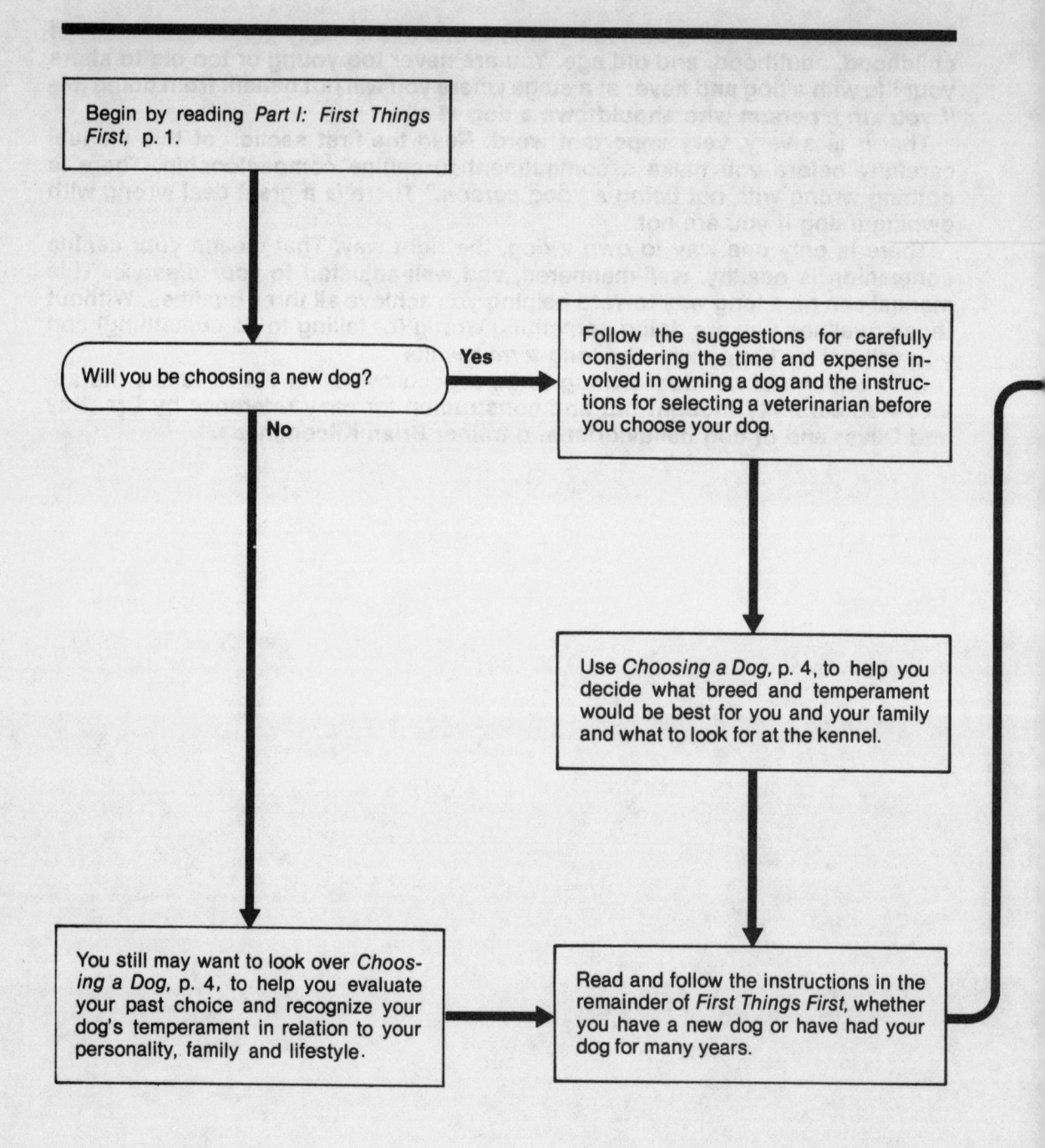

Begin by reading *Part I: First Things First*, p. 1.

Will you be choosing a new dog?

Yes → Follow the suggestions for carefully considering the time and expense involved in owning a dog and the instructions for selecting a veterinarian before you choose your dog.

Use *Choosing a Dog*, p. 4, to help you decide what breed and temperament would be best for you and your family and what to look for at the kennel.

No → You still may want to look over *Choosing a Dog*, p. 4, to help you evaluate your past choice and recognize your dog's temperament in relation to your personality, family and lifestyle.

Read and follow the instructions in the remainder of *First Things First*, whether you have a new dog or have had your dog for many years.

→ Turn to the *Strategy Chart: Health Problems & Emergency Care,* p. 44. Read and follow the instructions on avoiding some health problems and what to do should others arise. → Begin housebreaking, teething and chewing intervention, and basic obedience training as directed in the *Strategy Chart: Training Your Dog,* p. 16.

↓

Keep *Your Dog: An Owner's Manual* close at hand to use in the event of a training or health problem, or a medical emergency.

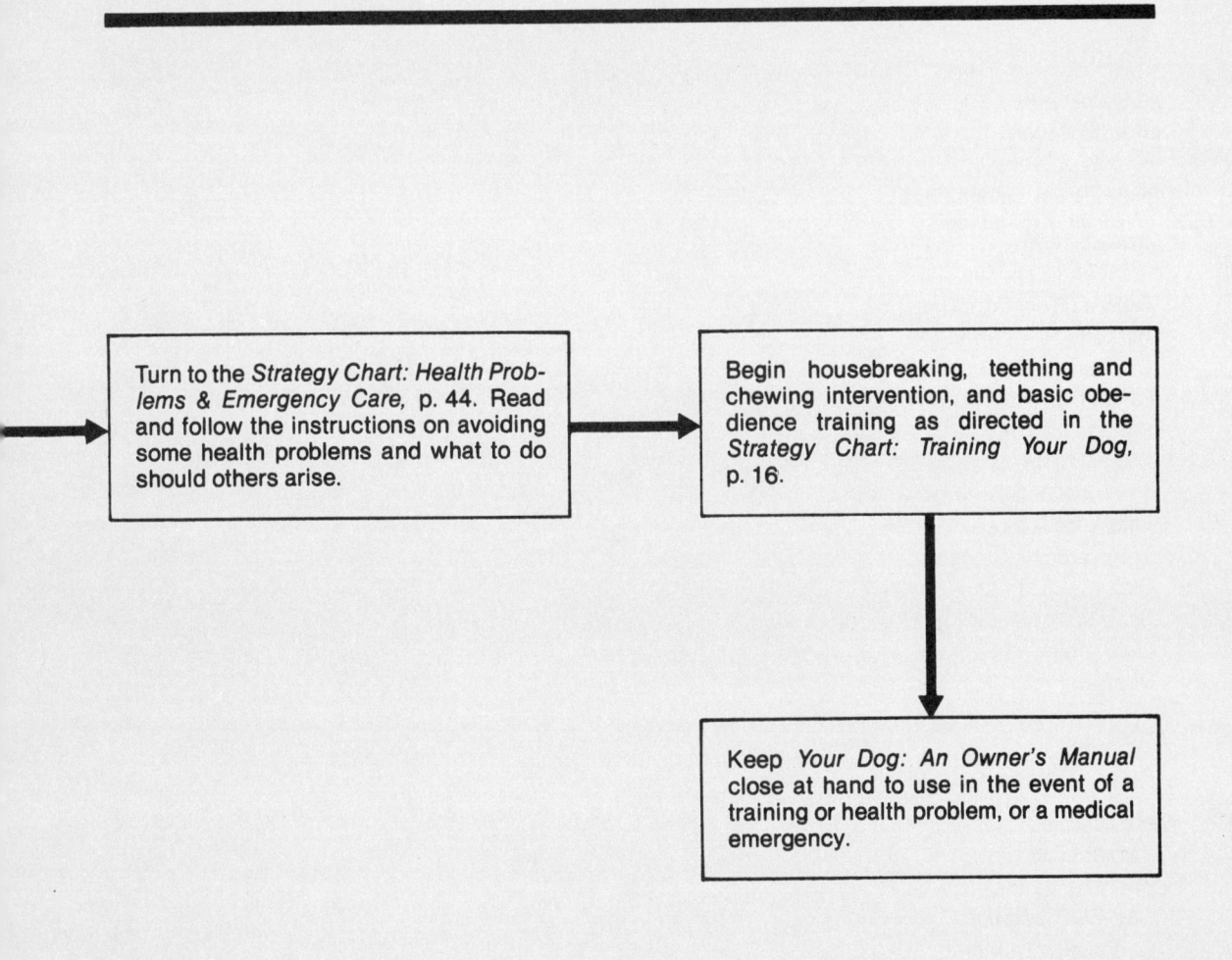

Contents

	Page
Emergencies	46
Health Record	i

Part I: First Things First

Introduction	2
Time and Expense	2
Before Choosing a Dog	2
Selecting a Veterinarian	3
Choosing a Dog	3
Choosing a Dog (Chart)	4
Picking the Breed and Temperament	8
Choosing the Age and Sex	8
Testing a Dog's Temperament	9
Immunizations and Worms	10
Transmittable Diseases	10
Diet	11
Spaying or Neutering	12
Grooming	12
Boarding Your Dog	13
Traveling with Your Dog	14

Part II: Training Your Dog

Introduction	18
Pack Instinct	18
Denning Instinct	19
Common Mistakes to Avoid	19
Choosing a Trainer	20
Brian Kilcommons Answers Some of the Most Frequently-Asked Questions about Dog Training	21

	See	
Abortion	Behavioral Emergencies	40
Barking	Problems	38
Begging	Obedience Training I	30
Behavioral Emergencies	Behavioral Emergencies	40
Biting or Nipping — emergency	Behavioral Emergencies	40
— non-emergency	Problems	38

viii

	See	Page
Boundary Training	Problems	38
Chasing People or Cars	Problems	38
Chewing	Teething & Chewing	28
Collars	Obedience Training II	32
Commands — part 1	Obedience Training I	30
— part 2	Obedience Training II	32
— part 3	Obedience Training III	34
— part 4	Obedience Training IV	36
Copulation	Behavioral Emergencies	40
Dog Fights	Behavioral Emergencies	40
Etiquette	Obedience Training I	30
Exercise — requirements	Choosing a Dog	4
— leash training	Obedience Training II	32
Fighting with Other Dogs	Behavioral Emergencies	40
Growling — emergency	Behavioral Emergencies	40
— non-emergency	Problems	38
Heeling	Obedience Training III	34
Housebreaking — general	Housebreaking	24
— problems	Problems in Housebreaking	26
Jumping on People or Furniture	Obedience Training I	30
Leash Training	Obedience Training II	32
Manners	Obedience Training I	30
"Mouthing"	Obedience Training I	30
Obedience Training — part 1	Obedience Training I	30
— part 2	Obedience Training II	32
— part 3	Obedience Training III	34
— part 4	Obedience Training IV	36
Paper Training	Housebreaking	24
Perimeter Training	Problems	38
Problems — barking	Problems	38
— begging	Obedience Training I	30
— biting	Problems	38
— chasing people or cars	Problems	38
— chewing	Teething & Chewing	28
— copulation	Behavioral Emergencies	40
— fighting with other dogs	Behavioral Emergencies	40
— growling	Problems	38
— housebreaking	Problems in Housebreaking	26

continued

Contents (cont.)

	See	Page
Problems — jumping on people or furniture	Obedience Training I	30
— "mouthing"	Obedience Training I	30
— nipping	Problems	38
— straying	Problems	38
— teething	Teething & Chewing	28
Socialization	Obedience Training I	30
Straying	Problems	38
Teething	Teething & Chewing	28
Walking — to housebreak	Housebreaking	24
— to leash train	Obedience Training II	32

Part III: Health Problems & Emergency Care
If there is more than 1 problem, turn to the most serious problem first.

Health Record		i
Introduction		50
Preventing Illness		50
When an Emergency Occurs		50
Taking Your Dog's Temperature		51
Giving Your Dog a Pill		52
Giving Your Dog Liquid Medication		52
Pregnancy		52
Euthanasia		53

	See	
Emergency Principles	Basic Emergency Principles	56
Medical Supplies	Basic Medical Supplies	54
Moving the Seriously Injured Dog	Back & Neck Injuries	78
Moving the Sick or Injured Dog	Transporting to Veterinarian	58

Lifesaving Procedures

Artificial Respiration	Artificial Respiration & CPR	60
Choking	Choking	62
Drowning	Artificial Respiration & CPR	60
Heart Massage	Artificial Respiration & CPR	60

Illnesses

Allergic Reaction — drug	Allergic Reaction	76

	See	Page
Allergic Reaction — food	Allergic Reaction	76
— insect sting	Insect Stings & Bites	88
— pollen	Allergic Reaction	76
Bleeding — anal	Diarrhea, Constipation & Anal Problems	68
— nasal	Nose Problems	92
Breathing Problems — absence of breathing	Artificial Respiration & CPR	60
— choking	Choking	62
— difficult breathing	Breathing Difficulties	64
— rapid breathing	Breathing Difficulties	64
— unconsciousness	Convulsions or Unconsciousness	66
Collapse	Convulsions or Unconsciousness	66
Constipation	Diarrhea, Constipation & Anal Problems	68
Convulsions	Convulsions or Unconsciousness	66
Diarrhea	Diarrhea, Constipation & Anal Problems	68
Epileptic Seizures	Convulsions or Unconsciousness	66
Fever	Fever	70
Gastrointestinal Problems	Diarrhea, Constipation & Anal Problems	68
Nasal Discharge	Nose Problems	92
Nosebleed	Nose Problems	92
Parasites — internal	Diarrhea, Constipation & Anal Problems	68
— external	Insect Stings & Bites	88
Sneezing	Nose Problems	92
Swelling	Swelling	98
Unconsciousness	Convulsions or Unconsciousness	66
Vomiting	Vomiting	72
Worms	Diarrhea, Constipation & Anal Problems	68

Accidents & Injuries

Abdominal Injury	Abdominal & Chest Injuries	74
Abrasion	Minor Cuts & Scratches	82
Amputation	Puncture & Deep Wounds	102
Back Injury	Back & Neck Injuries	78

continued

Contents (cont.)

	See	Page
Bleeding — abdominal	Abdominal & Chest Injuries	74
— chest	Abdominal & Chest Injuries	74
— deep wound	Puncture & Deep Wounds	102
— eye	Eye Injuries	84
— minor wound	Minor Cuts & Scratches	82
— mouth	Tooth & Mouth Injuries	100
— nose	Nose Problems	92
Burns	Burns	80
Chemical Burn — eye	Eye Injuries	84
— body	Burns	80
Chest Injury	Abdominal & Chest Injuries	74
Choking	Choking	62
Collapse	Convulsions or Unconsciousness	66
Convulsions	Convulsions or Unconsciousness	66
Cut — minor	Minor Cuts & Scratches	82
— serious	Puncture & Deep Wounds	102
Drowning	Artificial Respiration & CPR	60
Electric Shock	Burns	80
Eye Injury	Eye Injuries	84
Facial Injury	Head & Facial Injuries	86
Foreign Object — abdomen	Abdominal & Chest Injuries	74
— anus	Diarrhea, Constipation & Anal Problems	68
— chest	Abdominal & Chest Injuries	74
— eye	Eye Injuries	84
— foot	Swelling	98
— mouth	Choking	62
— nose	Nose Problems	92
— throat	Choking	62
Head Injury	Head & Facial Injuries	86
Jaw Injury	Head & Facial Injuries	86
Leg — injury	Leg Fractures, Sprains & Dislocations	90
— wound	Puncture & Deep Wounds	102
Mouth Injury	Tooth & Mouth Injuries	100
Neck Injury	Back & Neck Injuries	78
Nosebleed	Nose Problems	92
Paralysis	Back & Neck Injuries	78

	See	Page
Puncture Wound	Puncture & Deep Wounds	102
Scratch	Minor Cuts & Scratches	82
Smoke Inhalation	Artificial Respiration & CPR	60
Tooth Injury	Tooth & Mouth Injuries	100
Unconsciousness	Convulsions or Unconsciousness	66
Wound — minor	Minor Cuts & Scratches	82
— serious	Puncture & Deep Wounds	102

Poisoning, Bites & Stings

Animal Bites — minor	Minor Cuts & Scratches	82
— serious	Puncture & Deep Wounds	102
Bee Sting	Insect Stings & Bites	88
Chemical Burns	Burns	80
Chemical Poisoning	Poisoning	94
Chiggers	Insect Stings & Bites	88
Fleas	Insect Stings & Bites	88
Food Poisoning	Poisoning	94
Fumes — inhaled	Poisoning	94
Insect Sting	Insect Stings & Bites	88
Parasites — internal	Diarrhea, Constipation & Anal Problems	68
— external	Insect Stings & Bites	88
Poisoning — ingested or inhaled	Poisoning	94
Scorpion Bite	Insect Stings & Bites	88
Snakebite	Snakebite	96
Spider Bite	Insect Stings & Bites	88
Tick — embedded	Insect Stings & Bites	88
Wasp Sting	Insect Stings & Bites	88

Exposure to Heat or Cold

Cold Exposure	Cold Exposure & Frostbite	104
Frostbite	Cold Exposure & Frostbite	104
Heat Exhaustion	Heatstroke & Heat Exhaustion	106
Heatstroke	Heatstroke & Heat Exhaustion	106
Hypothermia	Cold Exposure & Frostbite	104

1
FIRST THINGS FIRST

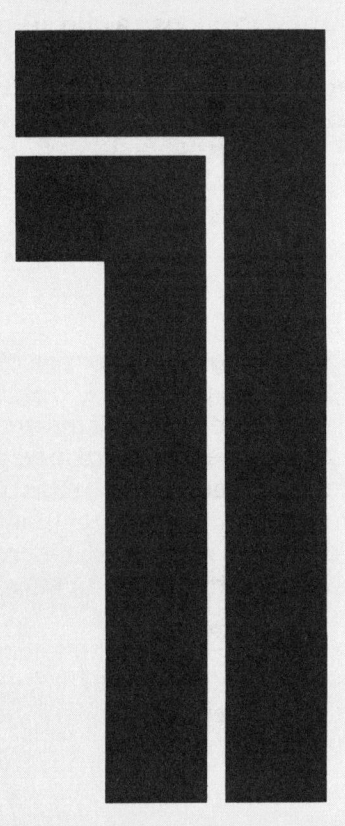

Part 1
Introduction

Your Dog: An Owner's Manual is a total care manual for your dog. The first half of the manual will help you decide how to choose a dog, if you don't already have one, and how to care for and train him. The second half will help you deal with medical problems and emergencies you may encounter as a dog owner — everything from fractures and choking to nosebleed and vomiting.

Time and Expense

Before you decide whether getting a dog is wise for you or your family, consider the time and expense of ownership. Besides feeding and watering, he will need to be walked several times a day and exercised often. Time and patience are needed for training, instilling good habits, and preventing bad ones. And these are just the fundamentals of dog ownership. A dog also needs a great deal of love and companionship — essentially, unpressured time from you and other humans. In many ways, owning a dog is like having a child — you will be responsible for all of his basic needs. But unlike a child, he won't grow up and learn to care for himself; you will need to provide for him for the rest of his life.

The expense of fulfilling these needs — food, shelter, collars and leashes, routine and unexpected veterinary visits, and perhaps training — add up to quite a bit of money. You should be aware of the expenses involved in owning a dog and be ready to assume them before you commit yourself.

Before Choosing a Dog

Before you choose a dog, learn what his basic exercise and grooming requirements are and whether or not the breed you prefer would be a wise choice for you or your family. The charts on pp. 4-7 will help you decide this. In addition, know what you will be feeding him, the basic rules of the house he will be expected to obey, who your veterinarian will be, and where the dog will be kept until he is housebroken; in essence, prior to selecting a dog, skim this book and read this introductory section carefully. In addition, make certain that any family members, *including* children, are aware of all decisions you make.

Children must know how to care for the dog, but a young child cannot — and should not — be given the total responsibility. Training is an essential part of dog ownership, and this responsibility cannot be turned over completely to a child. In addition, children must learn early how to handle a dog properly — never striking, yelling, pinching, or intimidating him, and certainly never pulling his tail, ears, or paws. As explained later (see p. 10), a dog will justifiably protect himself against injury.

Selecting a Veterinarian

Your veterinarian is your partner; together it is your responsibility to keep your dog physically healthy. When you get a dog, you should have already chosen a veterinarian, after carefully researching several in your area. Ask friends, neighbors, and your breeder for recommendations. Make an appointment with one or two of those suggested and ask to see their facility. A veterinarian who refuses your request is probably not a good choice. Look for a confident veterinarian with a clean facility. Be sure to find out:
— what days and hours the veterinarian practices
— what care is provided after office hours
— what other services, such as grooming and bathing, are available
— if there is X-ray equipment on the premises.

Choosing a Dog

Choosing a new dog is not as simple as picking the cutest or most amusing puppy in a litter from your favorite breed. A puppy that seems playful and happy may grow up to be too assertive or energetic for you, your lifestyle, or your family. A breed that's right for your neighbor may not be right for you. When you are choosing a dog, remember that a healthy dog's personality, or temperament, can fall into three basic categories:
— *Low dominance:* placid, sedate, and easygoing, but not shy or insecure.
— *Medium-to-high dominance:* active, playful, and outgoing, but not as assertive as some others.
— *High dominance:* assertive, protective, strong-minded and in need of an assertive and confident master or mistress.

Shy or insecure dogs do not have healthy temperaments and generally will not make good pets. These dogs often hide or crouch when approached, and while they may seem cute, their basic insecurity can lead to many problems, including biting. Your personality and whether or not you have children play key roles in choosing both the breed of dog and the temperament of the dog that's best for you. While temperament is a factor to consider in picking a breed of dog, choosing between puppies in that breed and finding one with the appropriate temperament for you is also important. Even within one litter temperaments vary, sometimes ranging from shy to overly assertive.

Choosing a Dog

You will notice that some breeds appear in several categories. The reason is that there are temperament differences within breeds. It is important that you use the temperament tests on p. 9 to judge a specific dog's disposition.

If you are . . .	By temperament tests, look for a dog who is . . .
A family with one or more young children	Low in dominance Placid Easy-going Not "mouthy"
A family with older children	Medium-to-high in dominance Active Happy Out-going
A reactive person	Low in dominance Placid Easy-going

key: ▲ good watchdog ● requires daily grooming ● requires a great deal of exercise
◐ requires frequent grooming ◐ requires moderate exercise
○ requires minimal grooming ○ requires minimal exercise

Consider these breeds:	watchdog	grooming	exercise
Basset Hound		○	○
Bearded Collie	▲	●	◐
Bichon Frise		●	◐
Cairn Terrier	▲	◐	◐
Collie	▲	●	●
Corgi		○	◐
English Springer Spaniel		◐	●
Golden Retriever		◐	●
Jack Russell Terrier	▲	○	●
Labrador Retriever	▲	○	●
Newfoundland		●	○
Shih Tzu		●	○
Standard Poodle	▲	●	◐
West Highland White Terrier		◐	◐
Afghan Hound		●	●
Airedale	▲	◐	●
Alaskan Malamute		◐	●
Basset Hound		○	○
Boxer	▲	○	●
Collie	▲	●	●
English Setter		◐	●
English Springer Spaniel		◐	●
Golden Retriever		◐	●
Great Dane	▲	○	●
Irish Setter	▲	◐	●
Jack Russell Terrier	▲	○	●
Labrador Retriever	▲	○	●
Long- or Wirehaired Dachshund	▲	●	◐
Old English Sheepdog	▲	●	◐
St. Bernard	▲	◐	◐
Siberian Husky		◐	●
Smooth Dachshund	▲	○	◐
Standard or Giant Schnauzer	▲	●	●
Basset Hound		○	○
Bulldog		○	○
Collie	▲	●	●
English Setter		◐	●
Labrador Retriever	▲	○	●
Mastiff	▲	○	○
Newfoundland		●	○
St. Bernard	▲	◐	◐

continued

Choosing a Dog (cont.)

You will notice that some breeds appear in several categories. The reason is that there are temperament differences within breeds. It is important that you use the temperament tests on p. 9 to judge a specific dog's disposition.

If you are . . .	By temperament tests, look for a dog who is . . .
A previous dog owner who is assertive and confident and wants and can handle a protective, assertive dog	High in dominance Protective Assertive
A previous dog owner who wants an active, happy, outgoing dog	Medium-to-high in dominance Active Happy Out-going
An easy-going person	Medium-to-high in dominance Active Happy Out-going

key: ▲ good watchdog ● requires daily grooming ● requires a great deal of exercise
◐ requires frequent grooming ◐ requires moderate exercise
○ requires minimal grooming ○ requires minimal exercise

Consider these breeds:	watchdog	grooming	exercise
Akita	▲	◐	◐
Alaskan Malamute		◐	●
Bouvier des Flandres	▲	◐	●
Briard	▲	◐	●
Chesapeake Bay Retriever	▲	◐	●
Doberman Pinscher	▲	○	●
German Shepherd	▲	◐	●
Giant Schnauzer	▲	●	●
Jack Russell Terrier	▲	○	●
Long- or Wirehaired Dachshund	▲	●	◐
Rottweiler	▲	◐	●
Smooth Dachshund	▲	○	◐
Afghan Hound		●	●
Airedale	▲	○	●
Basset Hound		○	○
Beagle		○	●
Boxer	▲	○	●
Golden Retriever		◐	●
Jack Russell Terrier	▲	○	●
Labrador Retriever	▲	○	●
Long- or Wirehaired Dachshund	▲	●	◐
Old English Sheepdog	▲	●	●
St. Bernard	▲	◐	◐
Smooth Dachshund	▲	○	◐
Afghan Hound		●	●
Airedale Terrier	▲	○	●
Boxer	▲	○	●
Cairn Terrier	▲	○	◐
English Springer Spaniel		◐	●
German Shorthaired Pointer	▲	○	●
Golden Retriever		◐	●
Jack Russell Terrier	▲	○	●
Labrador Retriever	▲	○	●
Long- or Wirehaired Dachshund	▲	●	◐
Newfoundland		●	○
Old English Sheepdog	▲	●	●
Scottish Terrier	▲	◐	◐
Smooth Dachshund	▲	○	◐
Soft-Coated Wheaten Terrier	▲	●	●
Toy Poodle	▲	●	○
West Highland White Terrier	▲	○	◐
Yorkshire Terrier	▲	●	◐

Picking the Breed and Temperament

First, look over the chart on pp. 4-7 and read through the "If you are . . ." column. If you have children, this will take precedence over any other factor. If you have no children, choose the category that best describes *you*. Look at the description of the temperament, and the choice of breeds best suited to you. In choosing between these breeds select ones that fit into your lifestyle. The symbols next to each breed can be interpreted through the key at the top of each page. They will help you choose or eliminate breeds based on the amount of training, exercise, and grooming they require. The symbols also help identify breeds that are known for being good watchdogs.

Once you have narrowed the possible breeds down to two or three, do some outside research. Find out everything you can through friends, acquaintances, clubs, dog magazines, shows, and books before deciding on one breed.* Ask about the life expectancy of dogs of the breeds you have chosen and if they are known for being particularly hard to housebreak. Get to know several dogs in each breed, if possible. While you are researching, learn what to look for when choosing a dog from each breed and the names of a *good* breeder for each one. While puppies in many pet stores are well cared for, many are sent across the country in small cages — a practice that can lead to housebreaking and temperament problems. Also, picking a dog from a pet store gives you no opportunity to meet the breeder and see the parents of the puppy.

An inexpensive way to obtain a dog is through adoption from a local animal shelter (dog pound or humane society, etc.). You should be aware that there may be housebreaking and temperament problems similar to those encountered with pet shop puppies, but these may be solved through immediate housebreaking and obedience training intervention as discussed in Part II. The temperament tests on p. 9 can help you to avoid choosing a dog with a severe personality problem.

Choosing the Age and Sex

Many people wanting a pet overlook the older dog, believing it is always best to start off with a puppy. Older dogs are the most difficult to place in homes, but people should realize that older dogs offer many advantages. With older dogs size is known, looks are established, personality is formed, and they are usually housebroken. Potential owners who do not want to go through the chewing and housebreaking problems associated with puppies can find a perfect alternative in an older dog.

Deciding between a male and a female dog is a personal preference, but other factors must be taken into consideration. Females are smaller in size, go into

---

*There are several excellent comprehensive guides to the breeds. A number of authorities recommend *The Roger Caras Dog Book*, by Roger Caras (Holt, Rinehart and Winston, New York City, $16.95).

season twice a year, are less likely to roam, and are generally more submissive than males. First-time owners and people looking for an easier dog to live with might be happier with a female. Spaying will eliminate the problem of the female dog going into heat. Males are generally larger, have a higher aggression level, and are more likely to compete with their owners for control. Unless altered, they have a tendency to roam.

Testing a Dog's Temperament

When you go to the kennel (or kennels, if at all possible), do not be hasty in making a decision. Remember that you will be caring for and living with the dog for the rest of his or her life. This is an important decision that should not be rushed or left to children. You will need to screen not only each puppy, but the owner and the puppy's parents as well. A good breeder will be screening *you* at the same time, to be sure he is choosing an appropriate home for his puppy.

Before viewing the puppies, ask to observe the parents away from the litter. Although the father may not be available, it is important to see at least the mother. The puppy's parents should be happy and interested in being with you. Ask the owner to let the mother loose, away from the litter. It is not a good sign if she backs away and won't allow you to pet her; a dog in her litter will not be a good one for you to choose, because temperament is hereditary, and her puppies are likely to be insecure also. Consider visiting another kennel; a good breeder can breed most, if not all, insecurity out of his lines.

If the mother is happy and allows you to pet her, observe the puppies for several minutes to try to determine the level of dominance. The breeder should be able to help you when the dominance level is not obvious, and the following tests also will aid you in selecting the puppy with the appropriate temperament.

— Throw a ring of keys into the den. Those puppies that run up to investigate are more secure than those who look curious but don't venture forward.

— Cradle each puppy in your arm as you would a baby, with the stomach up. Rule out any puppies that try to right themselves. Place your hand between the front legs on the chest, and rule out any that tightly grab your hand with their paws.

— One by one, take the puppies to a room. Place the puppy on one side of the room and walk to the other side. Although it is good if a puppy follows you to the other side, it is best to give the puppy this "opposite sides" test: Squat and clap your hands; a puppy who is confident and outgoing will come to you with head and tail raised and an alert expression; a puppy who is alert but lower in dominance and not as secure as his outgoing sibling will come to you somewhat more slowly with his head down and his tail wagging. Often this type of puppy will lie down and roll onto his back to expose his stomach in a submissive position. A puppy who is shy, insecure, or aloof will not come

to you and may simply stare. It is best to rule out that puppy and any who run to the corner or crouch.
— If you have children, test the puppies for sensitivity of skin. Although most dogs will justifiably protect themselves when children pull their tails, ears, or legs, a good way to cut down on potential problems is to test each dog by gently pinching him on his side near his stomach. If he turns to snap at you, he will not make a good dog for children. Dogs differ in their skin sensitivities, and the puppy who snaps is not necessarily a "good" or "bad" dog; he simply is not a good choice for children.

Before making a final decision, be sure the puppy is physically healthy and meets standards for the breed as well as can be determined at this point in the dog's life. Ask for a money-back guarantee in case the dog becomes sick within 48 hours after you buy him or evidences a serious temperament problem. Ask about hereditary diseases and other problems such as trick knees, monorchism (having an undescended testis), and entropion eyes (the turning inward of the edge of the eyelid). Ask to see certificates ruling out hip dysplasia (abnormal growth of the hip) in both parents.

Immunizations and Worms

Your dog will need to visit the veterinarian several times as a puppy and yearly after the first year. Dogs require a number of vaccinations, and keeping them up-to-date will protect your dog from serious illnesses such as distemper, hepatitis, leptospirosis, and rabies. Regional and seasonal preventive medication, such as that for heartworm and parvovirus diarrhea, also may be necessary. The veterinarian, like your own physician, will keep a medical file for your dog, but it is a good idea to fill in the health record chart inside the front cover of this book so you will have a quick reference. Be sure to keep any medical records provided by the breeder or previous owner to avoid double vaccinations and cut down on costs.

Periodic examinations for worms should be included in the routine visits to the veterinarian. However, be alert to any discomfort your dog may be experiencing, and have him evaluated whenever you suspect worms. The chart *Diarrhea, Constipation & Anal Problems*, p. 68, will help you decide if symptoms need to be assessed.

Transmittable Diseases

There are several potentially serious disorders that can be transmitted to humans from dogs — sometimes through another agent — including:
— Tick-, deerfly-, and/or horsefly-transmitted diseases such as Rocky Mountain spotted fever and tularemia. Check your dog, yourself, and your family periodically for

ticks. When removing a tick, do not handle it with your bare hands, and never crush it; after removal, burn it. (See p. 88.) If you or a family member develop headache, chills, fever, or a rash and you have reason to suspect contact with a tick, deerfly, or horsefly, seek medical care immediately.

— Roundworm infestation. Although sometimes there are no symptoms in humans infested with roundworms, an infected person may experience abdominal pain and/or diarrhea. The infestation has the potential of being quite dangerous, particularly if the eye or brain is affected. To prevent transmission, have your dog evaluated as soon as you suspect worms. Keep areas your dog has soiled clean, and do not allow children to play in these areas.

If your dog was not wormed within a few weeks after birth, assume he has roundworm and have him evaluated and treated by your veterinarian as soon as possible.

— Hookworm infestation. Characterized by welts and itchy hands, feet, and other exposed surfaces, hookworm infestation may not be serious. However, it is an unpleasant experience. To prevent it — as you would when you suspect roundworms — have your dog evaluated at the first suggestion of worms. Keep areas where your dog has soiled clean, and do not allow children to play in these areas, particularly when they are barefooted.

— Heartworm infestation. While your dog cannot give you heartworm, the same mosquitos that can infect your dog can infect you. Although generally there are no symptoms associated with heartworm infestation and it is not serious in humans, a heartworm lesion in the lung can fool a physician and result in unnecessary and costly procedures for the patient. If your doctor detects a lesion in your lung and you suspect it may be related to heartworm because your dog has (or other dogs in your area have) — or had — heartworm, be sure to tell him. To protect your dog from heartworm, give the preventive medicine prescribed by your veterinarian as directed.

Diet

Your veterinarian can also help you select your dog's diet. There are three basic forms of food sold commercially: canned, semi-moist, and dry. Ask your veterinarian which form or combination of forms is best for your dog. Most dog-food packages recommend the amount to give. Be sure to choose brands that are properly balanced in carbohydrates, proteins, fats, and minerals. In addition:

— If you want to offer table scraps, ask your veterinarian what amounts and combinations will assure adequate nutrition. Keep in mind that pregnant or lactating dogs, puppies, dogs who require a large amount of exercise, and those who live outdoors during the cold months usually need more protein in their diets. Supplementing the diet with protein-rich cooked eggs, milk, fish, meat, or vegetables may be necessary; check with your veterinarian. Be sure the dog has plenty of water at all times. During

housebreaking, give water often, but only at specific times of the day. (See p. 24.)
— Give dog biscuits as treats or as rewards during training. Offer only one small biscuit each time, since you do not want treats to comprise a large part of your dog's diet; do not give biscuits to an overweight dog or one on a salt-restricted diet.
— If there is a chewing problem, you may want to give large, heavy shank bones to pacify the dog when he is left alone. (See *Teething & Chewing,* p.28.) However, giving animal bones is generally not recommended; if uncooked, grease can rub off on carpets and encourage the dog to chew the carpet, and cooked bones may splinter and cause injuries to the mouth. If splintering, cracked teeth, or other problems develop, keep bones away from the dog. Nylon bones *are* safe, and they will help keep a dog's teeth healthy.
— If your dog begins to gain or lose too much weight; develops a dull, dry coat; vomits; or has frequent diarrhea without other symptoms, be sure to contact your veterinarian. The problem may well be related to your dog's diet, and your veterinarian will decide whether to reduce or increase the amount of food. Remember, like that of humans, a dog's weight is determined by the food-exercise ratio. Many owners make the mistake of letting their dogs become overweight.

Spaying or Neutering

Any dog, except a purebred you intend to mate, should be spayed or neutered. Most of us would not hesitate to do this if we were aware of the number of dogs that are put to sleep each year because they cannot be placed in homes. The expense is well worth it: A bitch will no longer go into heat, and you will not need to worry about keeping her away from male dogs, and a male dog will not stray as far. People often worry about spaying or neutering causing weight gain and personality changes. However, there will be weight gain only if the proper food-exercise ratio isn't maintained, and any personality changes will only be for the better. Ask your veterinarian the age at which altering should be done, the cost, and what to expect. Taking your dog to an organization such as the local humane society that does low-cost spaying and neutering is an alternative.

Grooming

The amount of grooming and bathing required will depend largely on the breed. A short-haired dog will require little grooming, while other dogs may require daily grooming. Brush your dog's hair in one direction, and gently untangle knots or matting with a comb. The chart on pp. 4-7 shows the amount of grooming required by each of the more popular breeds. If you notice any skin irritation while grooming your dog,

contact your veterinarian. In addition:
— Bathe your dog only when needed.
— Different dogs have different kinds of coats; become familiar with the standard appearance of your dog's type. If your dog requires clipping, instead of paying for seasonal clips, you may want to make one appointment, watch how it's done, and clip him yourself from then on. The one-time expense will be a good investment, but be sure to ask as many questions as you can think of while you are at the grooming establishment.
— Clip your dog's nails as often as necessary. Nails require clipping when they become too long. For an indoor dog, this usually means about once a month; outdoor dogs usually require nail clipping less frequently. Ask your veterinarian to show you how to clip the nails properly.
— Have your dog's teeth cleaned during your yearly veterinary visits. If you notice an unusually bothersome mouth odor, green stains on the back teeth, or other signs of tooth decay or diseased gums, arrange to have a dental examination. Often the problem will not cause the dog pain, but it may lead to a serious disorder.
— Clean your dog's ears periodically to help prevent infection. Signs of ear infection include shaking of the head, scratching at the ears, and in later stages, a strong odor. Take a dog with these signs to the veterinarian as soon as possible. In the absence of infection or crusting, clean your dog's ears monthly or twice monthly, and after swimming or an outdoor trip, in this fashion: First, moisten the inside of each ear with an eyedropperful of mineral oil, gently clean with a cotton ball, then put a few drops of oil into the ear canal and remove wax and dirt with a cotton swab.
— If a skunk sprays your dog, saturate him with tomato juice to destroy the smell, then bathe him. For burns in the eye from the spray, see *Eye Injuries,* p. 84.
— If a substance, such as tar or chewing gum, becomes fixed in your dog's coat, keep the area moistened with mineral or vegetable oil about 8 hours, then wash with soap and water.

Boarding Your Dog

When you go away and decide not to take your dog with you, leave him in his home with a petsitter, if possible, or have a neighbor and/or friend feed, water, walk, and exercise him. If you must board your dog, shop around. Ask your veterinarian, friends, and neighbors for recommendations. If possible, visit the kennel ahead of time, looking for:
— clean, roomy cages with plenty of ventilation and light
— a view, whether the dog is indoors or out
— a run and an allocated amount of time each day for running
   Be sure to have your dog vaccinated against kennel cough and have all other immunizations updated, if necessary, two weeks before boarding.

Traveling with Your Dog

If you take your dog with you on a trip or move to a new home, avoid shipping him by plane or train, if at all possible; the stress of traveling alone can be very hard on a dog. Whatever mode of travel you use:
— Ask your veterinarian about motion sickness preventatives and tranquilizers.
— Check the rules and regulations pertaining to dogs with all airlines, railroads, ships, buses, hotels, and motels you will be using. Ask them for suggestions about making the trip as pleasant as possible for the dog. A booklet called "Touring with Towser," listing motels which allow dogs, is available from the Gaines Dog Research Center for $1.00.*
— If the dog will be traveling for more than a few hours, provide adequate food and water, and arrange for exercise. Adequate ventilation is imperative.

*"Touring with Towser," P.O. Box 1007, Kankakee, IL 60901.

2
TRAINING YOUR DOG

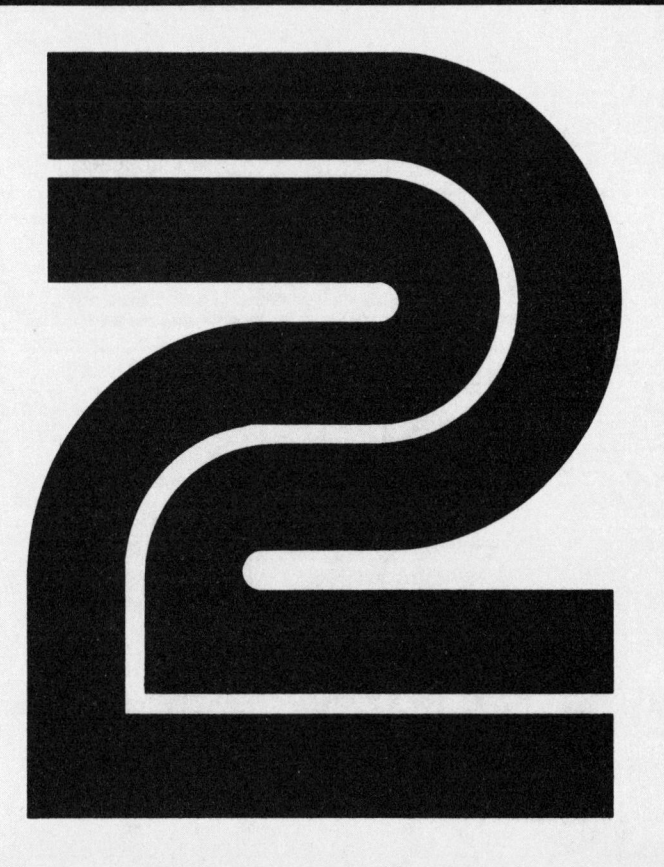

Strategy Chart: Training Your Dog

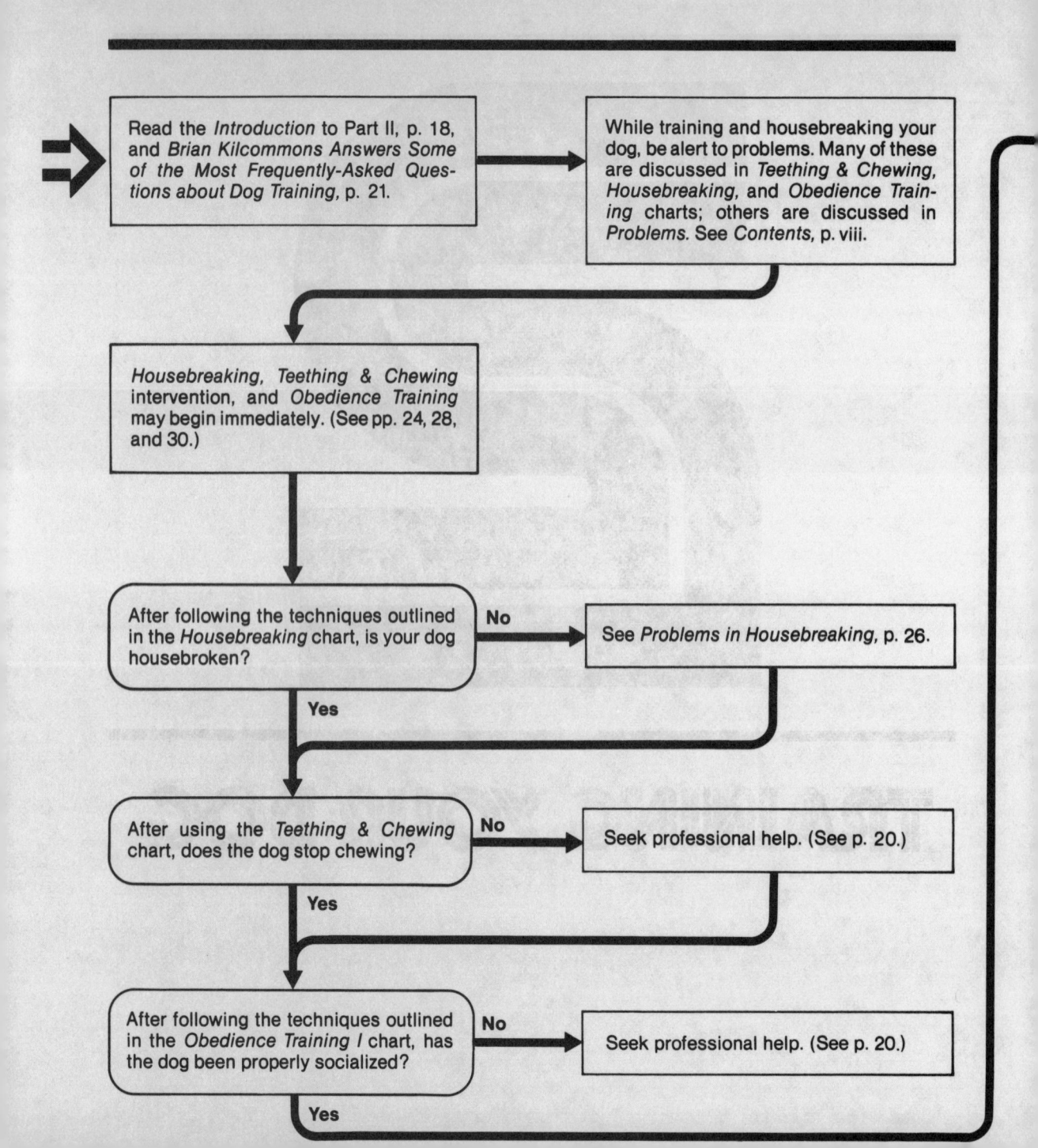

If a *Behavioral Emergency* occurs, see p. 40.

➡ Read the *Introduction* to Part II, p. 18, and *Brian Kilcommons Answers Some of the Most Frequently-Asked Questions about Dog Training*, p. 21.

While training and housebreaking your dog, be alert to problems. Many of these are discussed in *Teething & Chewing, Housebreaking,* and *Obedience Training* charts; others are discussed in *Problems*. See *Contents*, p. viii.

Housebreaking, Teething & Chewing intervention, and *Obedience Training* may begin immediately. (See pp. 24, 28, and 30.)

After following the techniques outlined in the *Housebreaking* chart, is your dog housebroken? — **No** → See *Problems in Housebreaking*, p. 26.

Yes

After using the *Teething & Chewing* chart, does the dog stop chewing? — **No** → Seek professional help. (See p. 20.)

Yes

After following the techniques outlined in the *Obedience Training I* chart, has the dog been properly socialized? — **No** → Seek professional help. (See p. 20.)

Yes

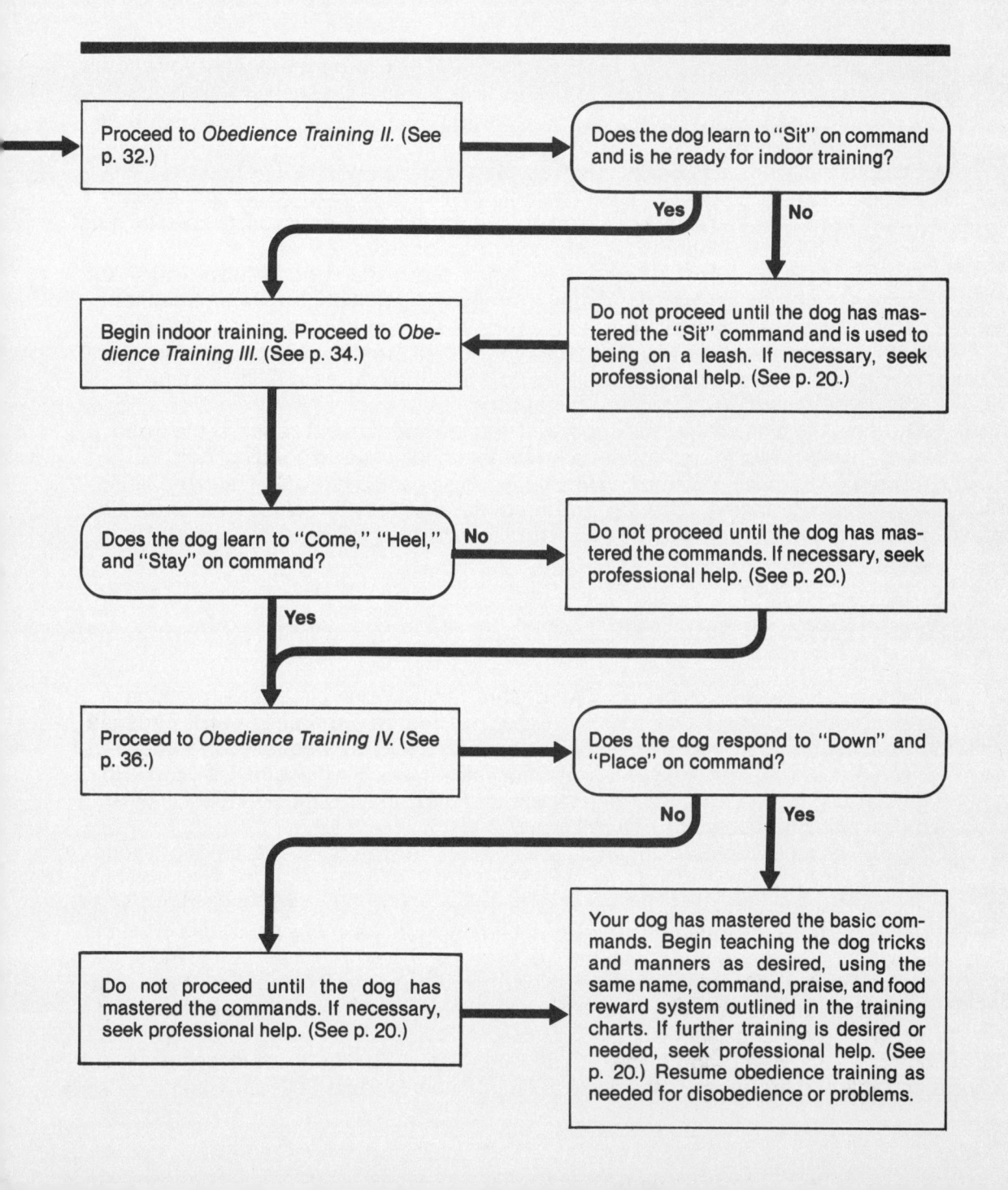

→ Proceed to *Obedience Training II.* (See p. 32.) → Does the dog learn to "Sit" on command and is he ready for indoor training?

- **No** → Do not proceed until the dog has mastered the "Sit" command and is used to being on a leash. If necessary, seek professional help. (See p. 20.)
- **Yes** → Begin indoor training. Proceed to *Obedience Training III.* (See p. 34.)

Does the dog learn to "Come," "Heel," and "Stay" on command?

- **No** → Do not proceed until the dog has mastered the commands. If necessary, seek professional help. (See p. 20.)
- **Yes** → Proceed to *Obedience Training IV.* (See p. 36.)

Does the dog respond to "Down" and "Place" on command?

- **No** → Do not proceed until the dog has mastered the commands. If necessary, seek professional help. (See p. 20.)
- **Yes** → Your dog has mastered the basic commands. Begin teaching the dog tricks and manners as desired, using the same name, command, praise, and food reward system outlined in the training charts. If further training is desired or needed, seek professional help. (See p. 20.) Resume obedience training as needed for disobedience or problems.

Part 2
Introduction

When the subject is dogs, everyone is an authority! Ask your friends what you should do about a canine-behavior problem and, in all likelihood, the answer will confuse you. Hit him, but not with your hand; use a newspaper as a club; rub his face in urine or excrement; knee him; lock him up; chain him; scream; plead; cry; beg; and so on.

Unfortunately, the advice of amateurs is almost always wrong. The homemade solutions create frustration in both dog and owner, and the original problems only worsen. In order for you to have both an obedient and happy dog, you, the owner, must understand his basic instincts and individual personality.

Training is teaching. No matter whom or what you are teaching, pain and intimidation make both your task and your pupil's unpleasant and difficult. Harsh treatment creates anxiety, promotes distrust, and can cause your dog to become aggressive. After you have created the learning problem yourself through your own (sorry!) ineptitude, you become convinced that your dog is too stupid to learn. That is a typical case history heard daily by professionals.

The biggest obstacle to achieving a well-trained dog, in most cases, is the owner's lack of correct information. An educated owner usually has an obedient dog.

Training is basically communication between dog and owner. Common problems, such as housebreaking, chewing, and jumping, can easily be solved if the proper information is available, first to the owner and then to the dog.

Pack Instinct

No other animal shares man's companionship, family, work, play, and protection to the degree the dog does. One reason the dog has adjusted so well to man is because he is descended from social animals. The hierarchy that is established in a wild dog or wolf pack is the instinct that guides and motivates the dog in its human-led pack. In each pack of dogs, one dog is the pack leader. This is usually the strongest, most intelligent animal, selected by nature to lead.

One of the most important instincts in a dog is to fit into a pack — to belong. If your dog is a born follower, your task isn't too difficult. If your dog is a born leader, you have some mutual adjustments to make. In order for you to be your dog's best friend, you must be his boss. No question about that; there are just too many situations in which the owner must be capable of making a decision and giving a verbal command to his "pack followers." Obedience by the dog is critical, because it establishes the owner as the dominant member of the pack. By establishing communication and teaching functional commands such as "Sit," "Come," "Down," "Heel," and "Stay," you take control. Your dog will know to look to you for direction. That puts you in the position of being able to direct verbally the dog's actions. If your leadership is consistent, your dog will be a pleasure to live with. Since most people will live with their dog for eight years or more, the sooner a dog understands what is expected of him, the better. The more you ask of your dog, the better he will respond to you, once the idea of pack leadership has been established as an element in both of your lives.

Denning Instinct

Housebreaking and chewing are the two problems most commonly reported by dog owners. Common sense and the use of your dog's instincts can help prevent or cure these problems.

Most dogs seek an enclosed or semi-closed area when they are tired or frightened. An area under a bed, chair, or table or in a corner is usually selected. Teaching a dog where his "den" is to be helps establish security and control, and problems with housebreaking and chewing are less likely.

Confine the dog to areas that allow enough room for him to lie down comfortably and turn around, but not large enough so that an "accident" can happen and be ignored. For example, a gate across the bathroom door makes a good enclosure. Never close the door, for most dogs will bark, chew, or scratch at the door to get out. Another solution is to use a crate as the enclosure.

Some of the most common mistakes are the result of the owner's over-reaction to a dog's behavior. Correcting with anger, instead of understanding, usually teaches a dog to react to you rather than to the situation. "I've hit him so many times, and he still does it over and over," owners often say, but there is a world of difference between *teaching* and *intimidation.* In order to teach your dog, you must be sure your dog is learning. Dogs crave attention, and at times negative attention is better than no attention at all. Consequently, if a dog is unable to get his owner's positive attention, he will try to get at least negative attention. Yelling and hitting are both forms of negative attention.

Common Mistakes to Avoid

Some basic rules to remember:
— Never yell at your dog. This shows a lack of control. Any response elicited from your dog will generally be out of fear or intimidation. The result will be inconsistent behavior and nervousness.
— Never hit your dog. This only teaches mistrust, and usually creates more problems.
— Be consistent in not allowing undesirable behavior, such as jumping on people or furniture or rushing to get out the door.
— Be consistent in enforcing commands. If you give a command, make sure the dog

obeys. Allowing a lapse in obedience even once in a while will encourage your dog to test you to see if you mean what you say.

— Never repeat a command without saying, "No!" first, once your dog knows his commands. Constantly repeating commands is like yelling "Fire!" when there is no fire. The first time people respond, but the second or third time they will wait to see if there really is a fire.

— Don't expect a dog to behave and respond like a person. One must understand the way a dog's instincts work and work with — not against — them. Also, remember that, like people, a dog has good and bad days, and on bad days, he should not be pushed too hard.

— Spend the time to learn how to teach your dog what is expected and what is proper behavior. Consider taking a course or getting individual instruction from a dog trainer as soon as possible. While this book sets down the basic principles and practices of dog training, the cost of professional help will be returned many times over. Always seek professional help when a problem becomes unmanageable.

Choosing a Trainer

To find a good obedience school, ask friends, relatives, your veterinarian, and your breeder for recommendations. Before choosing one, remember that there are different methods of dog training, and the first thing to do is to investigate the philosophy of the schools you are considering until you find the one that appeals to you. Secondly, within a particular methodology there are several individual schools, and here you must rely on meeting with the personnel to determine the schooling with which you feel most comfortable. Cost and lesson arrangements (i.e., in-the-home, group, or kennel) are other factors to evaluate.

— Brian Kilcommons

Brian Kilcommons Answers Some of the Most Frequently-Asked Questions about Dog Training

Q: I'm planning to get a puppy. Do you recommend paper training before housebreaking?

A: I am against paper training in principle, unless the owner wants the dog to relieve himself indoors or he must leave the dog alone for long periods. Paper training essentially tells the dog that it is all right for him to relieve himself indoors. When the time comes to teach him to go outside, the dog must then "un-learn" the behavior that you have been teaching him. It's confusing and frustrating for the dog, and time-consuming for you. Most dogs over four months old have developed sufficient control and can be housebroken within two weeks without paper training, if they are properly taught.

Q: My dog knows all of his commands and does not have a hearing problem, but sometimes I have to repeat myself 10-15 times before he listens. What am I doing wrong?

A: Repeating a command over and over only teaches your dog to ignore you. This is one of the most important principles of obedience training. A dog's hearing is 16 times more sensitive than ours, and he should not need more than one command, spoken in a normal tone of voice, to obey. If your dog doesn't respond to your first command, be sure that he has, in fact, learned the command. Then, if he doesn't obey the first time, tell him firmly, "No!" and then repeat the command. Never repeat the command in succession without a correcting "No!" in between commands. If the dog still doesn't obey immediately, administer a correction with the "No!". In the charts that follow, specific corrections are recommended for each common problem. After you administer a correction a few times, you'll find that to avoid your disapproval, the dog will obey on the first command.

Q: Is it possible that my dog is just plain dumb? I've tried just about everything to get him to behave, but nothing seems to work. Yet I see some dogs on the street who are models of obedience. What's the difference?

A: The difference may be the result of many things, including too much inbreeding, the distinctive rates at which some types of breeds seem to learn, or the dog's or your particular mood on a given day. But most likely, the problem is that you have not properly taught your dog, or you are not communicating with him in a way that he can understand and to which he can respond. Once you know the ways to "reach" him so that he knows what's expected of him, you'll find him much more responsive.

However, each dog is an individual, and it may take a while until you get to know him. Some highly sensitive dogs require only mild reprimands, while others need firmer corrections. You might also wish to check with your vet or dog trainer about your pet's diet, as this has been shown to affect a dog's behavior. Finally, never train your dog if he's not feeling well, or, on good days, for longer than 15-20 minutes (3-5 minutes for a puppy).

Q: I'm afraid to be stern with my dog. She's very sensitive and her feelings get hurt very easily, just like a person's. I don't want her to hate me. What should I do?

A: One of the greatest myths circulating today is the belief that because dogs are warm and friendly, they think and react just like people. Dogs are dogs, and although they make marvelous pets precisely because they are loving and sympathetic, they do not speak our language and do not react in logical, human ways.

Dogs have instincts and reflexes, and you must use these, not your emotions, to help show your dog what is expected of her. Rather than resent you for the correction, a dog will actually be relieved to know what pleases you, and what doesn't. Correction is not being unkind to your pet. Instead, it positions you correctly as the dominant member of the relationship, and builds your dog's respect for you.

Q: My family loves our new puppy, and we feel we can do a good job of training him on our own. He's been no problem so far, so why should we bother with dog obedience schools?

A: Knowing how you want your dog to behave and knowing how to teach him are two different things. Obedience training is not simply having your dog perform certain exercises or tricks; it represents a way of life between you and your dog. Whether or not you have the time to give your dog affection all day long, obedience training designates periods of time that you must spend alone with your pet. This attention — plus the feeling of pride and accomplishment your dog will have in being able to successfully perform for you — increases the amount of love and respect you will have for each other. It also puts you in total control of your dog. The result is a happier owner and a happier pet.

In fact, most veterinarians would agree with my recommendation of formal obedience training, not just in problem situations, but for all dogs. It's a sound investment — the emotional returns will last for years.

If you have any specific questions about your dog, you can contact Brian Kilcommons. His address is:

Brian Kilcommons
Kilcommons Professional Dog Training
24 Charter Avenue
Dix Hills, NY 11743

Housebreaking

Needed:
A shake can — Place 10-15 pennies in an empty, clean soda can and tape the top; the noise created when you shake the can at your side will distract a dog and make him discontinue unacceptable behavior.

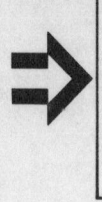

Until the dog is housebroken:
— Keep the diet consistent.
— Give no table scraps.
— Set the food down for 15 minutes; then give nothing to eat until the next scheduled meal, whether or not the last meal was eaten.

Confine the dog when left unsupervised until teething and housebreaking are completed (at about 6 months). Using toddler gates, a dog crate, or other barrier, create a "den" where the dog can be alone and take care of his basic needs, especially sleeping, eating, and drinking. Make the den only large enough to take care of his needs comfortably.

Are you at home most of the day?

Yes → Avoid paper training if at all possible, but it may be unavoidable with a dog purchased from a pet store or shelter. If necessary, place a thick layer of newspaper at one end of the den.

No → Is the dog less than 4 months old?

No → To housebreak the dog properly, walk him frequently. Give water before each walk and with each meal.
— If the dog is less than 4 months old, walk him before and after he eats, sleeps, chews on something, or plays, and when he sniffs around.
— If the dog is more than 4 months old, walk him *at least* 3 times a day.

Yes → Place a thick layer of newspaper at one end of the den on which he can relieve himself. Leave water when you're not going to be at home. Adjust the walking schedule as well as possible to your lifestyle.

When walking the dog:
— Say, "It's time to go out."
— Go to the same spot each time.
— Be sure he relieves himself before returning inside or playing with him, particularly during the last walk of the day.
— If necessary, walk him in an arc for stimulation. If this doesn't help, put him back in his den and walk him again after 15-30 minutes.
— During excretion, say, "Hurry up"; on completion, give praise and a food reward to teach him to excrete on command. After a week, begin to phase out rewards, giving one each time, then every two times, etc.

Never yell at or hit a dog, or rub his face in urine or excrement.

To clean up mistakes: Place several layers of paper towels on the urine or excrement. Pick up the feces, or absorb as much of the urine as possible. Wash the area with soap and water, trying not to spread the stain. On a linoleum or tile floor, scrub with water and ammonia, rinse, and let dry. On a carpet, scrub well with a solution of water and white vinegar, and blot dry. Sprinkle baking soda on the stain. After several hours, vacuum well. Commercial products may be used instead; follow label instructions.

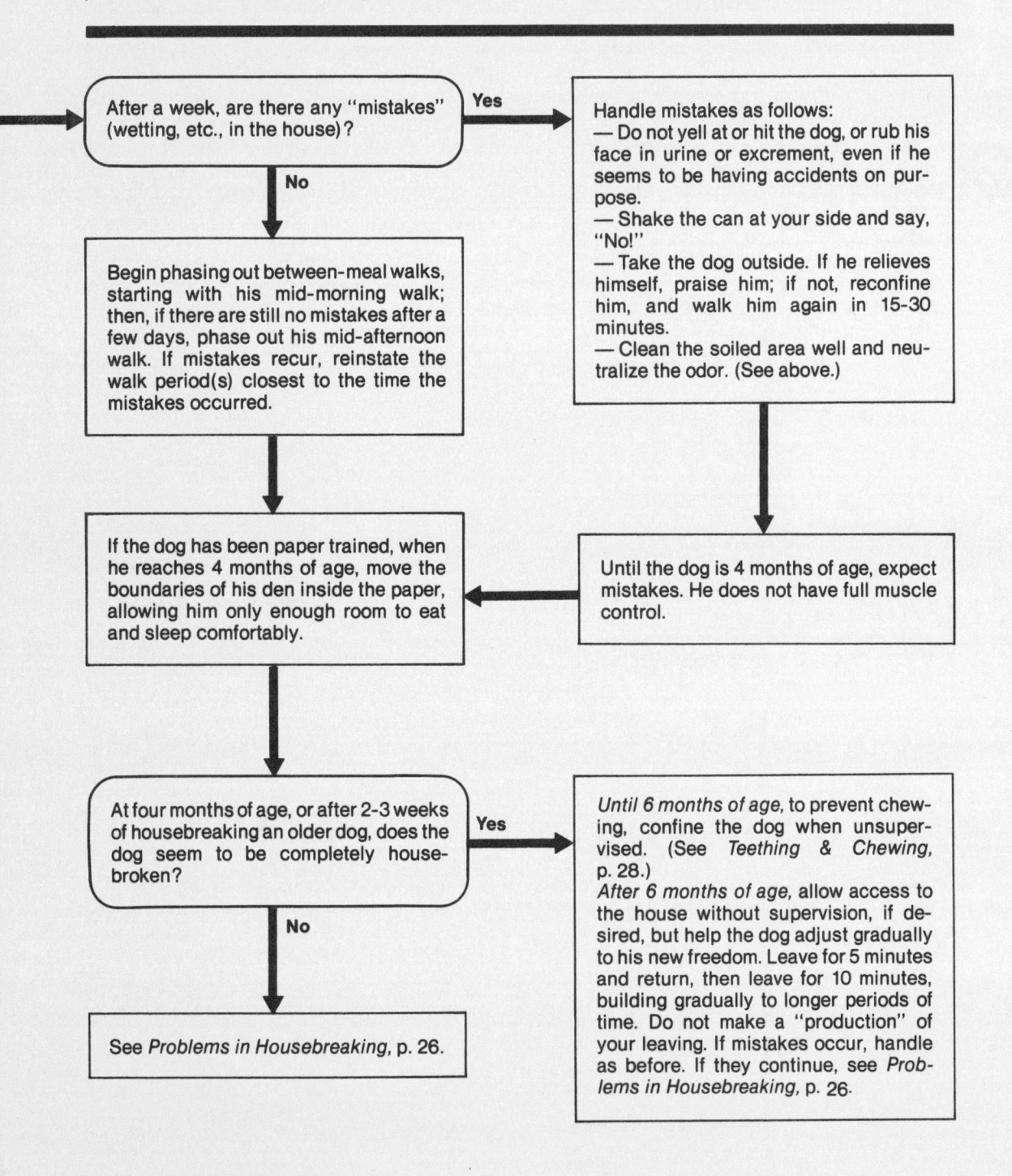

After a week, are there any "mistakes" (wetting, etc., in the house)? — **Yes** →

Handle mistakes as follows:
— Do not yell at or hit the dog, or rub his face in urine or excrement, even if he seems to be having accidents on purpose.
— Shake the can at your side and say, "No!"
— Take the dog outside. If he relieves himself, praise him; if not, reconfine him, and walk him again in 15-30 minutes.
— Clean the soiled area well and neutralize the odor. (See above.)

↓

Until the dog is 4 months of age, expect mistakes. He does not have full muscle control.

No ↓

Begin phasing out between-meal walks, starting with his mid-morning walk; then, if there are still no mistakes after a few days, phase out his mid-afternoon walk. If mistakes recur, reinstate the walk period(s) closest to the time the mistakes occurred.

↓

If the dog has been paper trained, when he reaches 4 months of age, move the boundaries of his den inside the paper, allowing him only enough room to eat and sleep comfortably.

↓

At four months of age, or after 2-3 weeks of housebreaking an older dog, does the dog seem to be completely housebroken? — **Yes** →

Until 6 months of age, to prevent chewing, confine the dog when unsupervised. (See *Teething & Chewing,* p. 28.)
After 6 months of age, allow access to the house without supervision, if desired, but help the dog adjust gradually to his new freedom. Leave for 5 minutes and return, then leave for 10 minutes, building gradually to longer periods of time. Do not make a "production" of your leaving. If mistakes occur, handle as before. If they continue, see *Problems in Housebreaking,* p. 26.

No ↓

See *Problems in Housebreaking,* p. 26.

Problems in Housebreaking

If the dog is less than 4 months old or is not housebroken, see *Housebreaking*, p. 24.

Never yell at or hit a dog, or rub his face in urine or excrement.

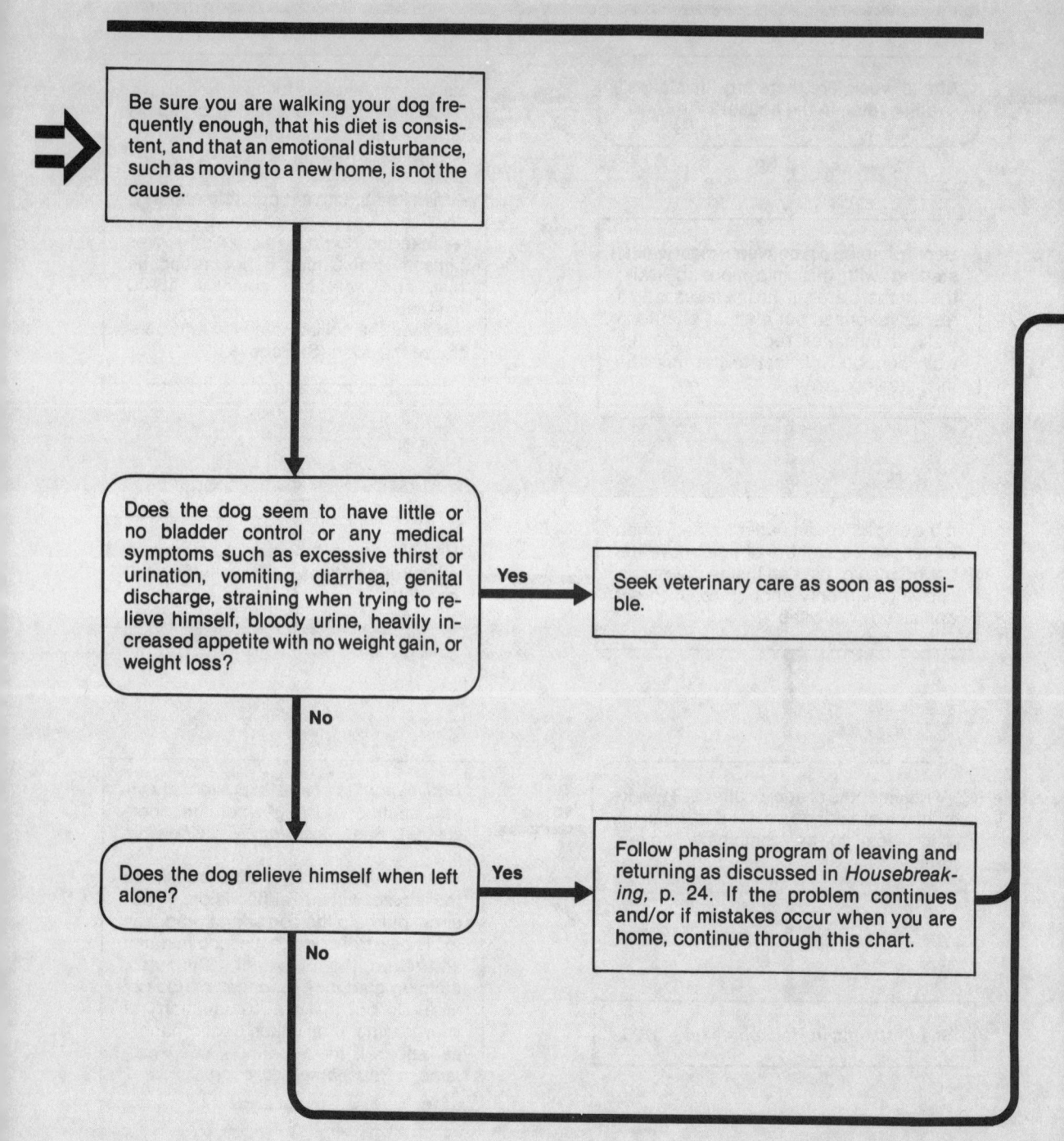

➡ Be sure you are walking your dog frequently enough, that his diet is consistent, and that an emotional disturbance, such as moving to a new home, is not the cause.

↓

Does the dog seem to have little or no bladder control or any medical symptoms such as excessive thirst or urination, vomiting, diarrhea, genital discharge, straining when trying to relieve himself, bloody urine, heavily increased appetite with no weight gain, or weight loss? — **Yes** → Seek veterinary care as soon as possible.

No ↓

Does the dog relieve himself when left alone? — **Yes** → Follow phasing program of leaving and returning as discussed in *Housebreaking*, p. 24. If the problem continues and/or if mistakes occur when you are home, continue through this chart.

No

To clean up mistakes: Place several layers of paper towels on the urine or excrement. Pick up the feces, or absorb as much of the urine as possible. Wash the area with soap and water, trying not to spread the stain. On a linoleum or tile floor, scrub with water and ammonia, rinse, and let dry. On a carpet, scrub well with a solution of water and white vinegar, and blot dry. Sprinkle baking soda on the stain. After several hours, vacuum well. Commercial products may be used instead; follow label instructions.

Start or advance *Obedience Training*. (See p. 30.) If the dog frequently urinates in particular rooms, practice obedience training in those rooms after all spots have been well cleaned and the odor neutralized. (See above.)

If the problem continues, the dog should be evaluated by a veterinarian to determine if a medical condition or the diet could be responsible. If these are ruled out, seek professional training help. (See p. 20.)

Teething & Chewing

Never yell at or hit a dog. Never play tug-of-war, or push his head from side-to-side, even playfully. These games will only teach him to be rough, probably rougher than you want. You — not your dog — know when "enough is enough."

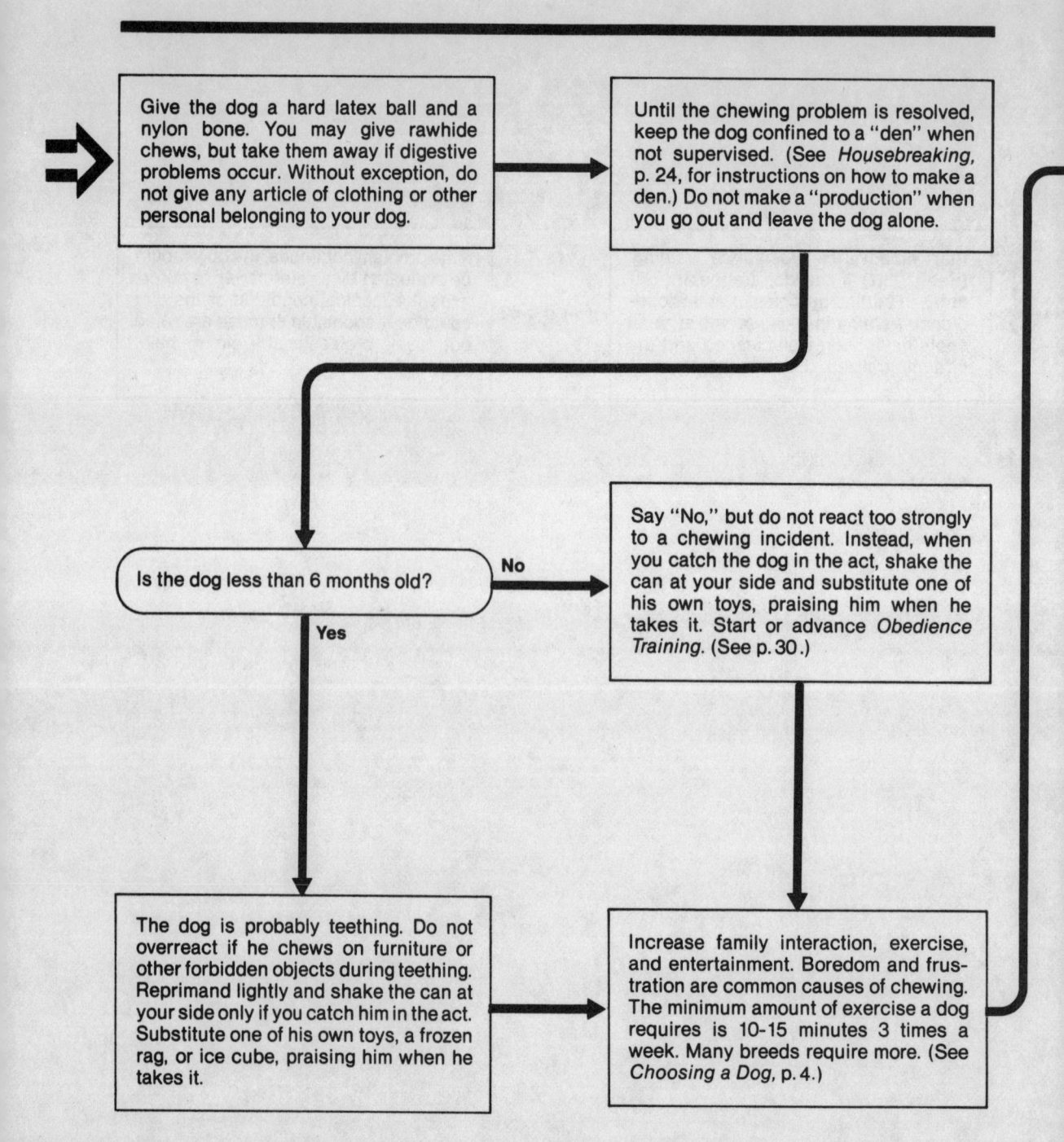

➡️ Give the dog a hard latex ball and a nylon bone. You may give rawhide chews, but take them away if digestive problems occur. Without exception, do not give any article of clothing or other personal belonging to your dog.

Until the chewing problem is resolved, keep the dog confined to a "den" when not supervised. (See *Housebreaking*, p. 24, for instructions on how to make a den.) Do not make a "production" when you go out and leave the dog alone.

Is the dog less than 6 months old?

No → Say "No," but do not react too strongly to a chewing incident. Instead, when you catch the dog in the act, shake the can at your side and substitute one of his own toys, praising him when he takes it. Start or advance *Obedience Training*. (See p. 30.)

Yes ↓

The dog is probably teething. Do not overreact if he chews on furniture or other forbidden objects during teething. Reprimand lightly and shake the can at your side only if you catch him in the act. Substitute one of his own toys, a frozen rag, or ice cube, praising him when he takes it.

Increase family interaction, exercise, and entertainment. Boredom and frustration are common causes of chewing. The minimum amount of exercise a dog requires is 10-15 minutes 3 times a week. Many breeds require more. (See *Choosing a Dog*, p. 4.)

Needed:
A shake can — Place 10-15 pennies in an empty, clean soda can and tape the top; the noise created when you shake the can at your side will distract a dog and make him discontinue unacceptable behavior.
Frozen rags — Freeze clean, damp rags for chewing to help dull the pain of teething when a dog is 4-6 months of age. Old washcloths or pieces of toweling are ideal.
Cheese bone — Boil a large, heavy shank bone to remove all grease, clean it out, and stuff it with American cheese. *Caution:* If splintering, cracked teeth, or other problems develop, discontinue immediately and seek veterinary care if necessary.

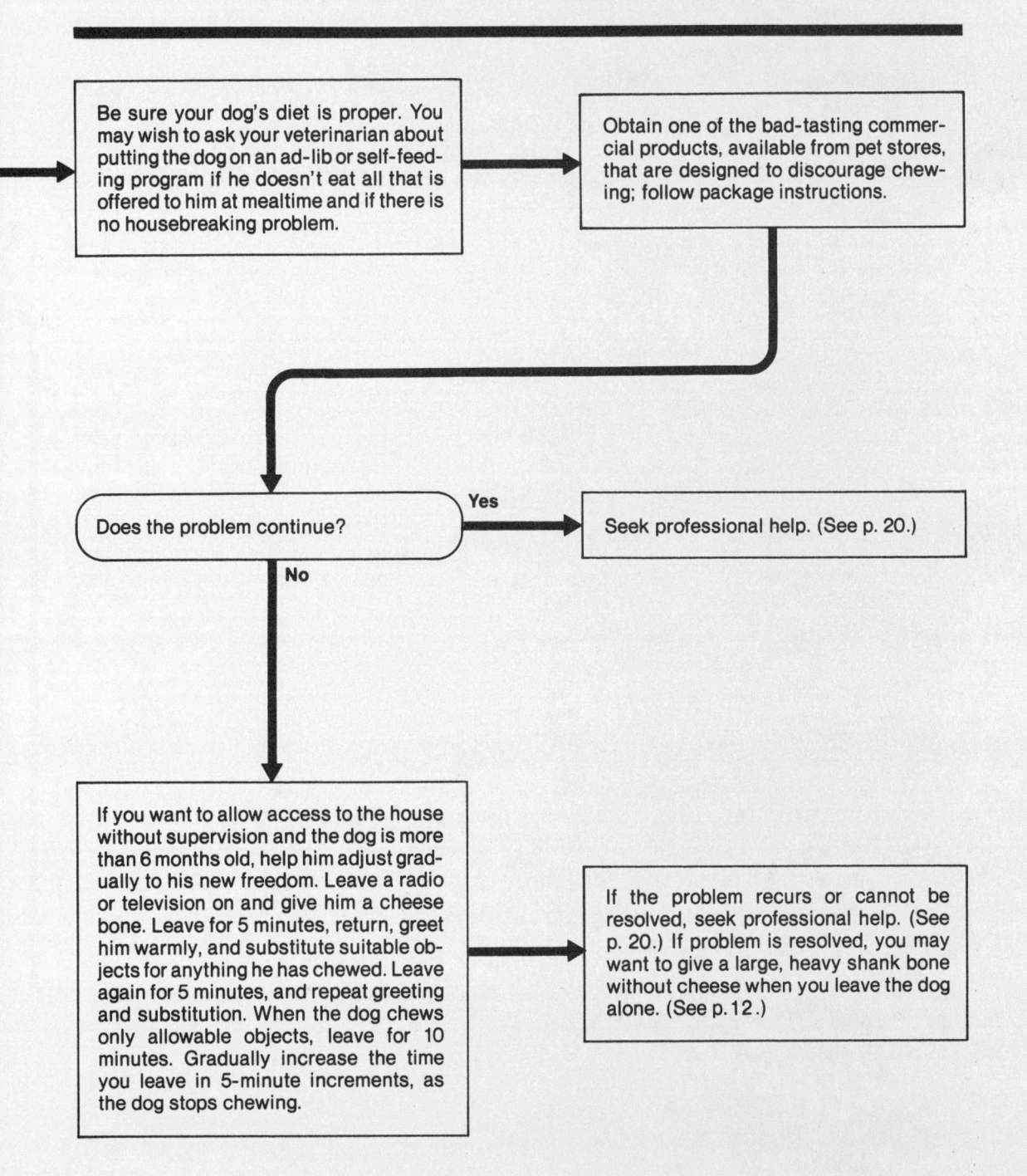

Be sure your dog's diet is proper. You may wish to ask your veterinarian about putting the dog on an ad-lib or self-feeding program if he doesn't eat all that is offered to him at mealtime and if there is no housebreaking problem.

Obtain one of the bad-tasting commercial products, available from pet stores, that are designed to discourage chewing; follow package instructions.

Does the problem continue? **Yes** → Seek professional help. (See p. 20.)

No

If you want to allow access to the house without supervision and the dog is more than 6 months old, help him adjust gradually to his new freedom. Leave a radio or television on and give him a cheese bone. Leave for 5 minutes, return, greet him warmly, and substitute suitable objects for anything he has chewed. Leave again for 5 minutes, and repeat greeting and substitution. When the dog chews only allowable objects, leave for 10 minutes. Gradually increase the time you leave in 5-minute increments, as the dog stops chewing.

If the problem recurs or cannot be resolved, seek professional help. (See p. 20.) If problem is resolved, you may want to give a large, heavy shank bone without cheese when you leave the dog alone. (See p. 12.)

Obedience Training I
(Including Etiquette, Manners & Socialization)

Needed:
A shake can — Place 10-15 pennies in an empty, clean soda can and tape the top; the noise created when you shake the can at your side will distract a dog and make him discontinue unacceptable behavior.

→ As soon as the dog has had all immunizations, take him frequently to public places, such as parks and shopping malls. Allow him to meet people and other dogs. Do not allow exceptions to behavior you are trying to teach him.

Never allow the dog to "mouth" you, or gnaw at you playfully. To prevent this, never push the dog's head from side to side or push him away from you.

Three important decisions to be made as soon as possible are whether you want to prevent your dog from:
— begging
— jumping on people
— jumping on furniture.

When the dog does mouth you, make as little movement as possible. Say, "No, leave." If he continues, shake the can at your side, say, "No" again, and give him one of his toys. If the problem continues, see *Teething & Chewing*, p. 28.

Do you want to keep your dog from jumping on people?

Yes → Squat when you pet the dog. When he jumps, shake the can at your side and say, "No." If he continues to jump, grab his front paws firmly. Continue to hold them when he cries — he is crying from frustration, not pain. Be consistent in not allowing him to jump, even if a visitor says, "I don't mind." If the jumping becomes a problem, seek professional help. (See p. 20.)

No → A dog cannot differentiate between when it is O.K. to jump and when it is not. While you and many visitors to your home may not mind, others might. You may wish to reconsider.

Socialization and etiquette are two of the most crucial parts of dog ownership. The best period for socialization is before the dog is 16 weeks old, but every dog should be socialized, and contrary to the old adage, you *can* teach an old dog new tricks. Dog etiquette, like human etiquette, helps make living with one another easier and is strongly encouraged. While the chart below applies to a new puppy, the principles may be applied to an older dog, whether he is new to the family or has been with you for many years.

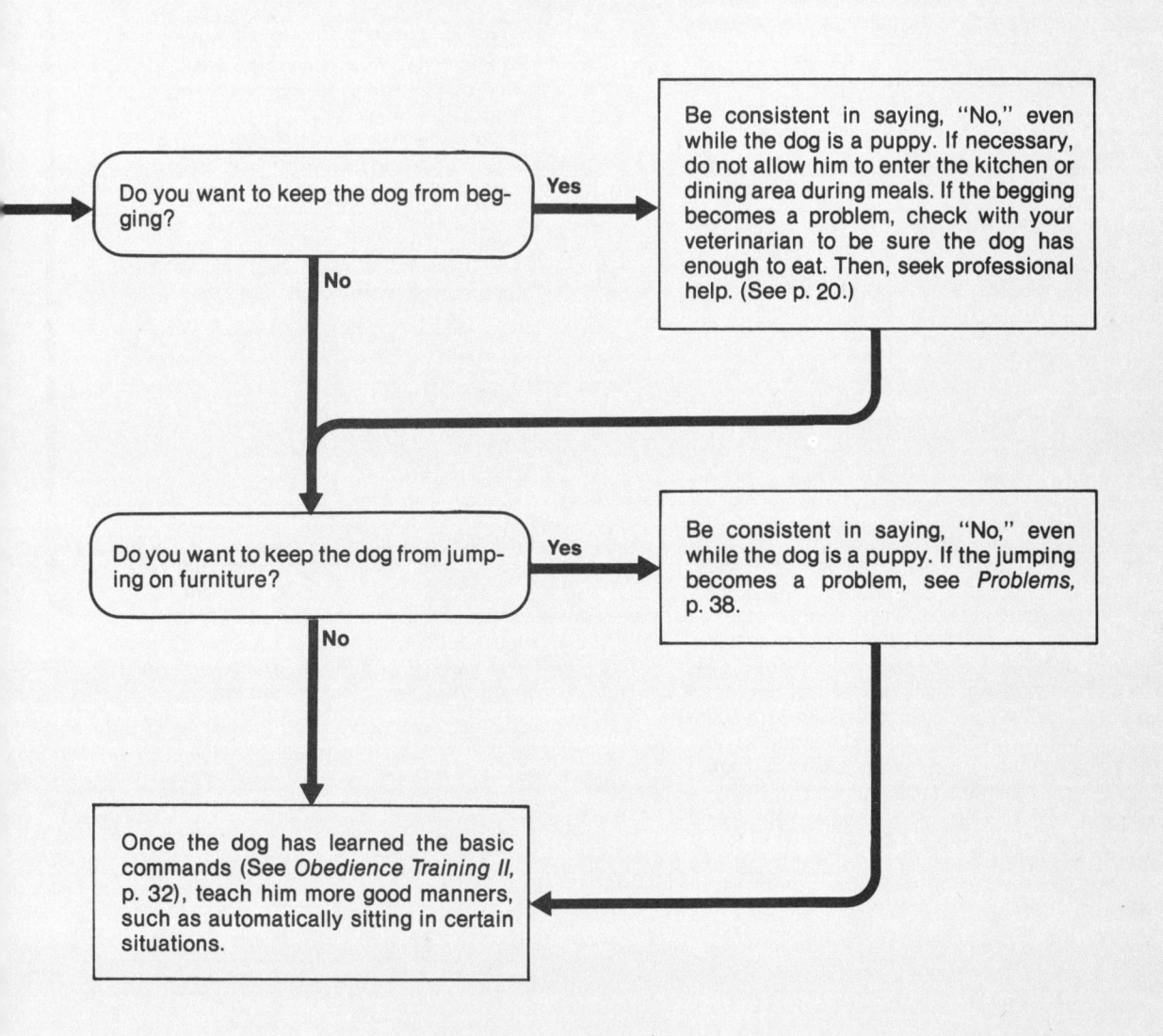

- Do you want to keep the dog from begging?
  - **Yes** → Be consistent in saying, "No," even while the dog is a puppy. If necessary, do not allow him to enter the kitchen or dining area during meals. If the begging becomes a problem, check with your veterinarian to be sure the dog has enough to eat. Then, seek professional help. (See p. 20.)
  - **No** ↓
- Do you want to keep the dog from jumping on furniture?
  - **Yes** → Be consistent in saying, "No," even while the dog is a puppy. If the jumping becomes a problem, see *Problems*, p. 38.
  - **No** ↓
- Once the dog has learned the basic commands (See *Obedience Training II*, p. 32), teach him more good manners, such as automatically sitting in certain situations.

Obedience Training II
(Including Basic Principles & Teaching "Sit")

Never yell at or hit a dog when he doesn't obey your command. Instead, reward him when he does obey with a lot of affection and a little food.

➡ Have the dog fitted with a choke collar at a pet store. Attach all immunization and license tags to the collar and put the collar on the dog.

➡ Practice training the dog for 6-8 weeks. The length of sessions *for a puppy* should be 3-5 minutes, 4-5 times a day, and *an older dog,* 15 - 20 minutes, 2-3 times a day. During training sessions:
— Always precede the command with the dog's name.
— Play a little with the dog during the training (once he has obeyed the particular command), and after training, but never allow him to gnaw at or "mouth" you or the leash.
— Train the dog initially in an area where there are no distractions.

➡ Once the dog has learned to obey a command, give it only once when directing him. If you are sure he knows the command, say, "No!" if he doesn't obey, and repeat the command. If the dog still doesn't obey immediately, say, "No!" again and use his collar or leash to give a short, sharp snap to let him know he is not responding appropriately. If the dog stops cooperating during a session, he may be tired. Make sure he completes the last command before you play with him.

➡ Teach the dog to sit. Say, "*(his name)*, sit," and scoop underneath his hindquarters while pushing the rear knees forward. When the dog sits in response to your command, give praise and a food reward. Practice this each time he is given a meal or taken outside.

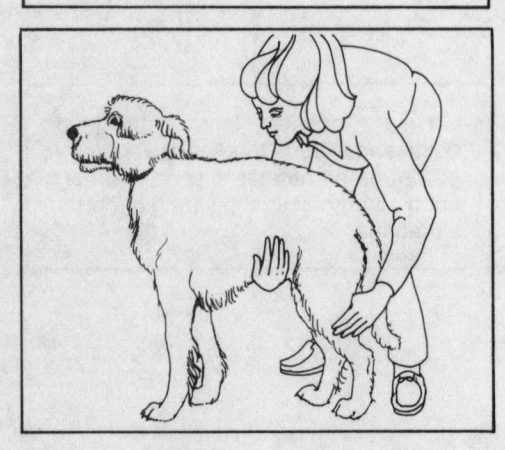

Needed:
A choke collar— Use a stainless steel chain collar with a ring at each end. Choke collars must be refitted as a dog grows. Do not use an electrical collar or a collar with spikes.
A training leash — Use a 6-foot leash made of canvas or leather.
A food reward —Give a dog biscuit or piece of cheese when your dog obeys a command.

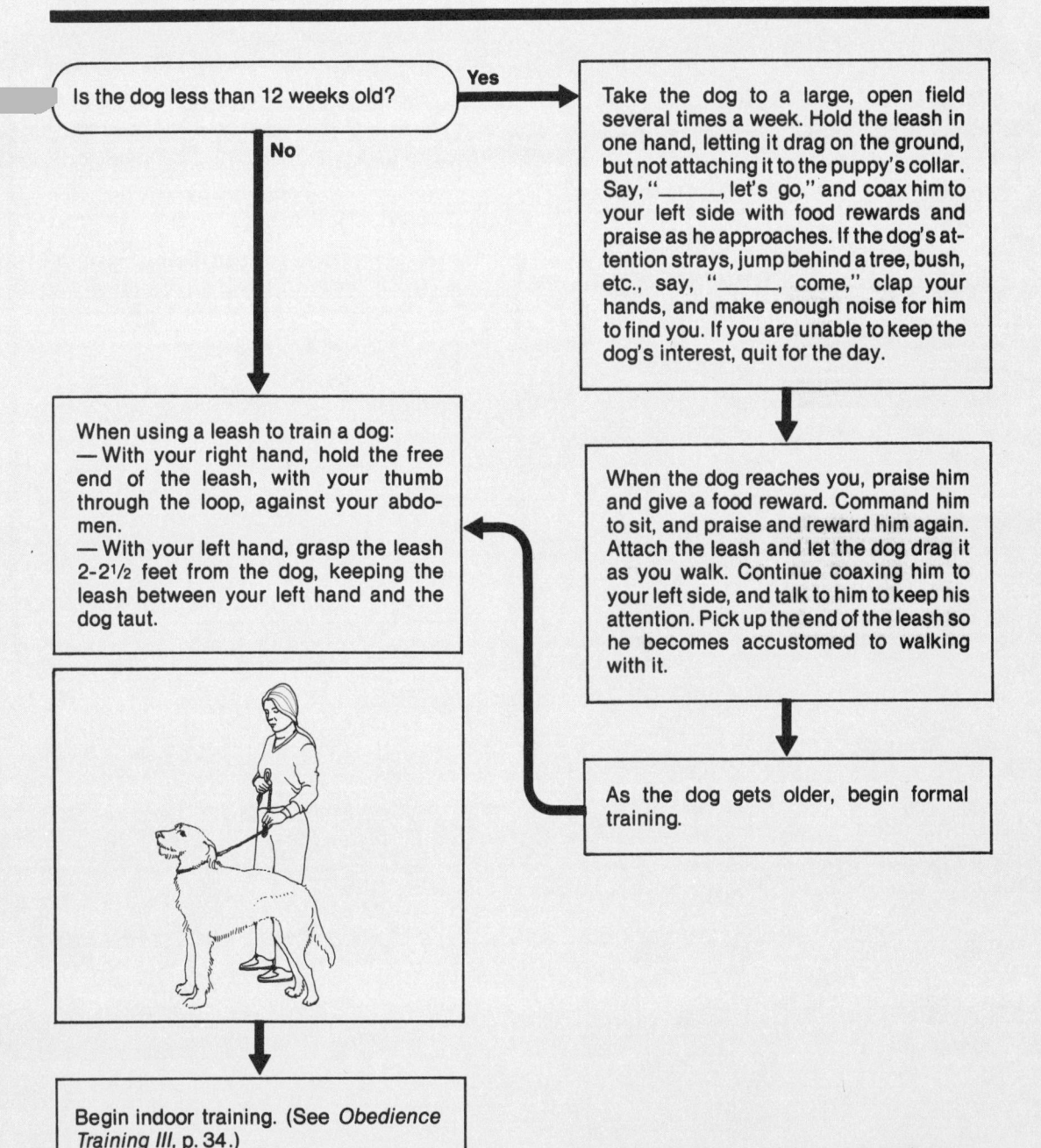

Is the dog less than 12 weeks old?

Yes → Take the dog to a large, open field several times a week. Hold the leash in one hand, letting it drag on the ground, but not attaching it to the puppy's collar. Say, "_____, let's go," and coax him to your left side with food rewards and praise as he approaches. If the dog's attention strays, jump behind a tree, bush, etc., say, "_____, come," clap your hands, and make enough noise for him to find you. If you are unable to keep the dog's interest, quit for the day.

When the dog reaches you, praise him and give a food reward. Command him to sit, and praise and reward him again. Attach the leash and let the dog drag it as you walk. Continue coaxing him to your left side, and talk to him to keep his attention. Pick up the end of the leash so he becomes accustomed to walking with it.

As the dog gets older, begin formal training.

No ↓

When using a leash to train a dog:
— With your right hand, hold the free end of the leash, with your thumb through the loop, against your abdomen.
— With your left hand, grasp the leash 2-2½ feet from the dog, keeping the leash between your left hand and the dog taut.

Begin indoor training. (See *Obedience Training III*, p. 34.)

Obedience Training III
(Including Teaching "Come," "Heel" & "Stay")

Never yell at or hit a dog when he doesn't obey your command. Instead, reward him when he does obey with a lot of affection and a little food.

The length of sessions *for a puppy* should be 3-5 minutes, 4-5 times a day, and *for an older dog*, 15-20 minutes, 2-3 times a day.

Begin indoor training with the dog on his leash. Squat and say, "_____, come," gently pulling the dog toward you if necessary. When he reaches you, give praise and a food reward and command, "_____, sit," praising and rewarding him again when he obeys. When the dog consistently responds to the "Come" command, move the training outdoors. Gradually increase the length of the leash (using clothesline) if the dog continues to obey.

Use the 6-foot leash to teach the dog to heel. With the dog at your left side, his head even with your leg, say, "_____, heel," and begin walking. Praise the dog throughout; do not allow him to get ahead of you or become distracted. If he does, give a short, sharp horizontal snap of leash and change direction.

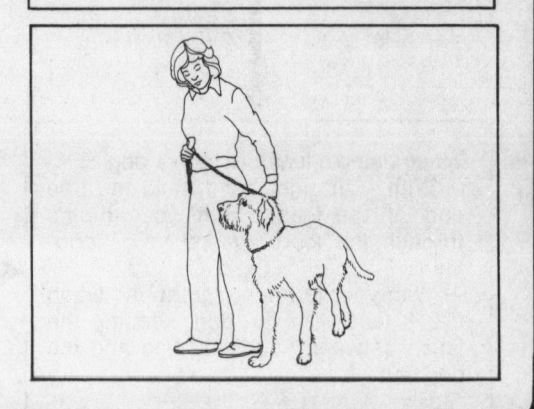

Walk the dog as before, then slowly stop and command him to sit at your left side. Say, "_____, stay," and simultaneously place your left hand, palm side down, in front of the dog's nose. Take the leash in your left hand again and slowly begin walking around the dog, stepping in front of him first, and keeping the leash at the right side of his head. Command the dog to sit and stay each time you stop heeling until it becomes automatic.

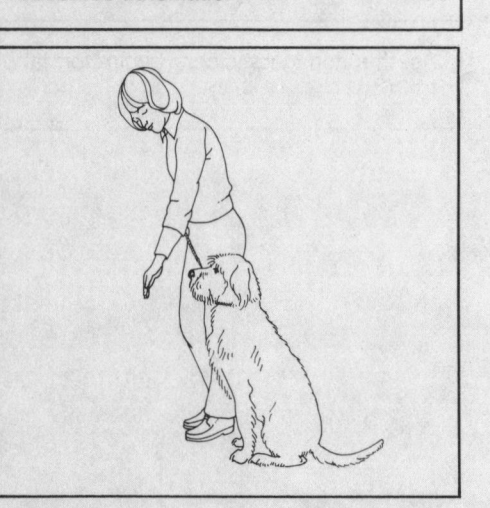

Needed:
A choke collar — Use a stainless steel chain collar with a ring at each end. Choke collars must be refitted as a dog grows. Do not use an electrical collar or a collar with spikes.
A training leash — Use a 6-foot leash made of canvas or leather.
A food reward — Give a dog biscuit or small piece of cheese when your dog obeys a command.

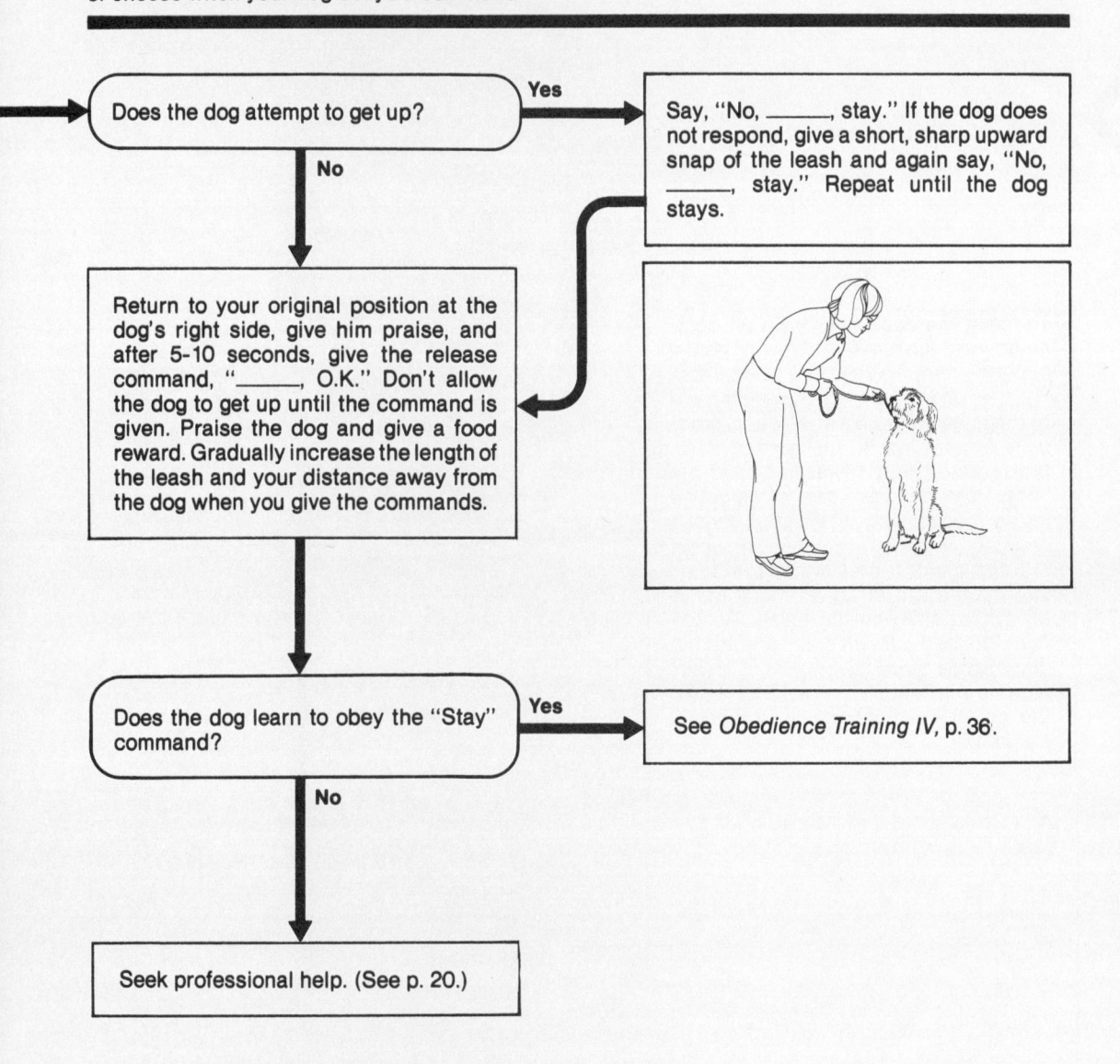

Does the dog attempt to get up? — **Yes** → Say, "No, _____, stay." If the dog does not respond, give a short, sharp upward snap of the leash and again say, "No, _____, stay." Repeat until the dog stays.

No ↓

Return to your original position at the dog's right side, give him praise, and after 5-10 seconds, give the release command, "_____, O.K." Don't allow the dog to get up until the command is given. Praise the dog and give a food reward. Gradually increase the length of the leash and your distance away from the dog when you give the commands.

Does the dog learn to obey the "Stay" command? — **Yes** → See *Obedience Training IV*, p. 36.

No ↓

Seek professional help. (See p. 20.)

Obedience Training IV

(Including Teaching "Down," "Place," & Tricks)

The length of sessions *for a puppy* should be 3-5 minutes, 4-5 times a day, and *for an older dog*, 15-20 minutes, 2-3 times a day.

➡ Give the dog the "Sit-stay" command. (See *Obedience Training III*, p. 34.)

To teach the dog to lie down on command, hold the leash in your right hand about 4 inches from the dog's neck, say, "_____, down," and use your left hand to press gently on his shoulders, gradually forcing him to the ground. Give praise and a food reward. Repeat the "Stay" command and give lavish praise and a food reward. If the dog doesn't respond, say, "No!" again, and repeat the command. If he still doesn't obey, say, "No!" again, and give a short, sharp downward snap on the leash. Be patient; this is a difficult command for the dog to obey since it puts him in a submissive position. After he has learned the command, continue to practice it frequently.

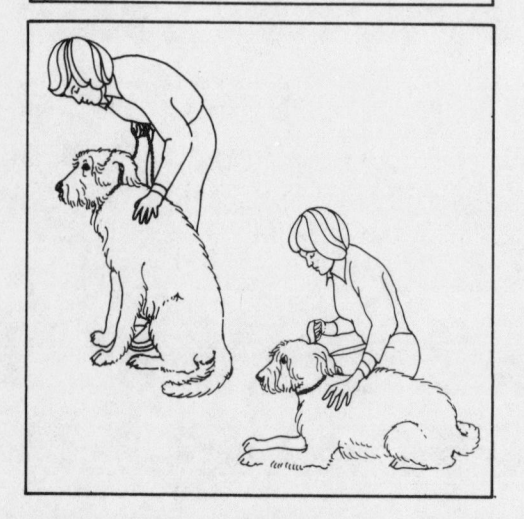

After 7 days of 2-3 training sessions per day, does the dog learn to obey the "Down" command?

Yes

No → Seek professional help. (See p. 20.)

Needed:
A choke collar — Use a stainless steel chain collar with a ring at each end. Choke collars must be refitted as a dog grows. Do not use an electrical collar or a collar with spikes.
A training leash — Use a 6-foot leash made of canvas or leather.
A food reward — Give a dog biscuit or piece of cheese when your dog obeys a command.

Never **yell at or hit a dog when he doesn't obey your command. Instead, reward him when he does obey with a lot of affection and a little food.**

Pick an area — or in a large house, several areas — in a corner or near a chair where the dog can be sent on command to be out of the way of family activities. With two pieces of food, lead the dog enthusiastically by his leash to the place and motion downward with one piece of food, saying, "____, place," until the dog lies down. The only command given is "____, place." Give praise and a food reward.

Walk a few feet away from the dog, and if he doesn't stay, say, "No!" and repeat the command. If he still doesn't respond, say, "No!" again and give short, sharp snaps of the leash horizontally to return him to the area, then downward to have him lie down. If or when he does stay, remove the leash and give praise and a food reward. Gradually increase the time period between the reward given for lying down and the reward given for staying. Use the "Place" command in the home or when visiting outside the home.

As the dog begins to learn the basic commands, begin practicing amid distractions, such as in a shopping center. As he learns to respond amid distractions, begin phasing out the food rewards, giving them every 2 times, then every 3, etc.

Once the dog has become obedient, use the same name, command, praise, and food reward system to teach tricks, such as shaking hands, playing dead, rolling over, and speaking, if desired. Obedience training should be resumed at the first sign of disobedience and is crucial in solving many common problems.

Problems

Never yell at or hit a dog.

Be sure the dog has had all immunizations.

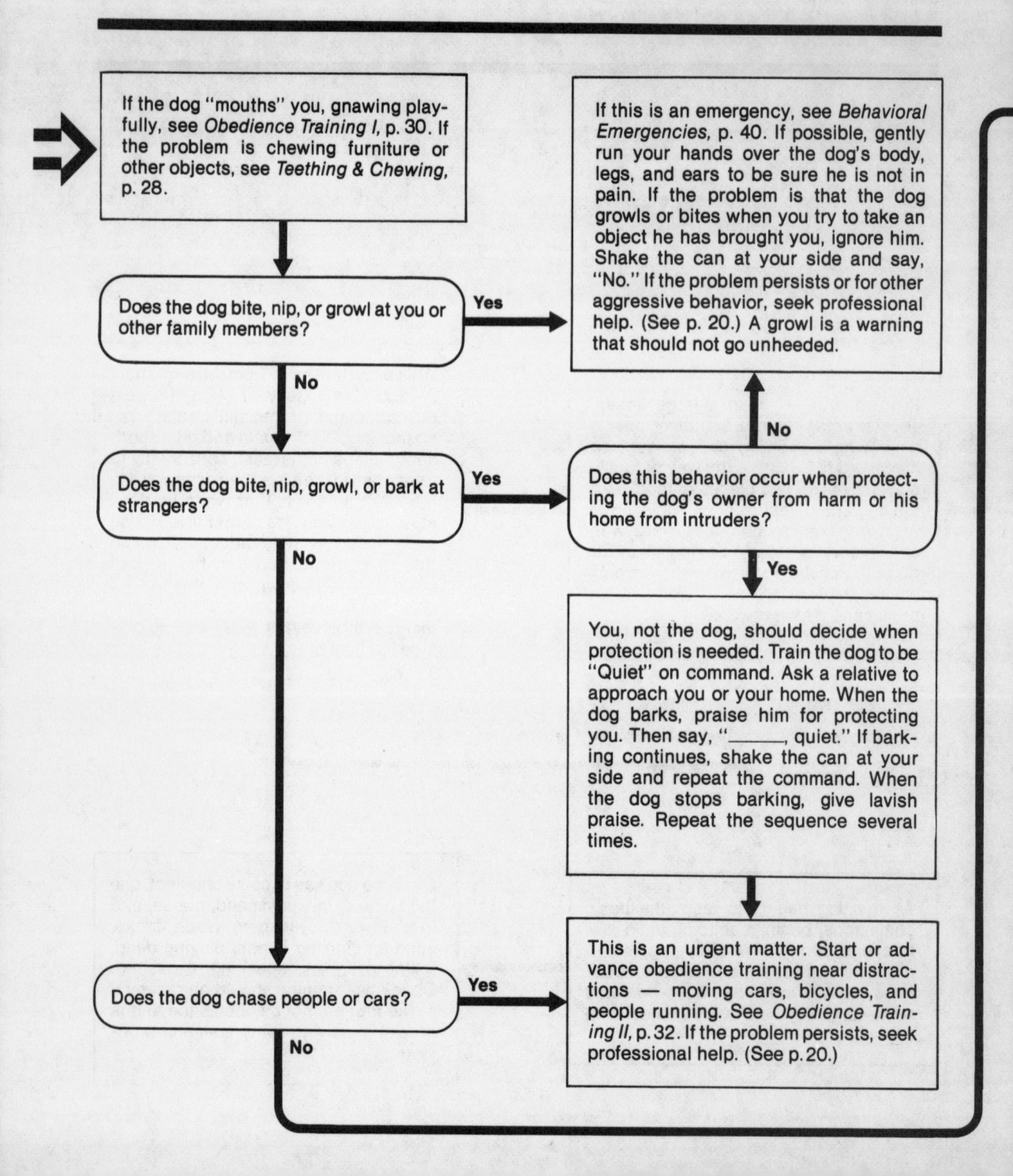

→ If the dog "mouths" you, gnawing playfully, see *Obedience Training I*, p. 30. If the problem is chewing furniture or other objects, see *Teething & Chewing*, p. 28.

↓

Does the dog bite, nip, or growl at you or other family members? — Yes → If this is an emergency, see *Behavioral Emergencies*, p. 40. If possible, gently run your hands over the dog's body, legs, and ears to be sure he is not in pain. If the problem is that the dog growls or bites when you try to take an object he has brought you, ignore him. Shake the can at your side and say, "No." If the problem persists or for other aggressive behavior, seek professional help. (See p. 20.) A growl is a warning that should not go unheeded.

↓ No

Does the dog bite, nip, growl, or bark at strangers? — Yes → **Does this behavior occur when protecting the dog's owner from harm or his home from intruders?**
— No ↑ (back to emergency box)
— Yes ↓

You, not the dog, should decide when protection is needed. Train the dog to be "Quiet" on command. Ask a relative to approach you or your home. When the dog barks, praise him for protecting you. Then say, "_____, quiet." If barking continues, shake the can at your side and repeat the command. When the dog stops barking, give lavish praise. Repeat the sequence several times.

↓ No

Does the dog chase people or cars? — Yes → This is an urgent matter. Start or advance obedience training near distractions — moving cars, bicycles, and people running. See *Obedience Training II*, p. 32. If the problem persists, seek professional help. (See p. 20.)

↓ No

Needed:
A shake can — Place 10-15 pennies in an empty, clean soda can and tape the top; the noise created when you shake the can at your side will distract a dog and make him discontinue unacceptable behavior.

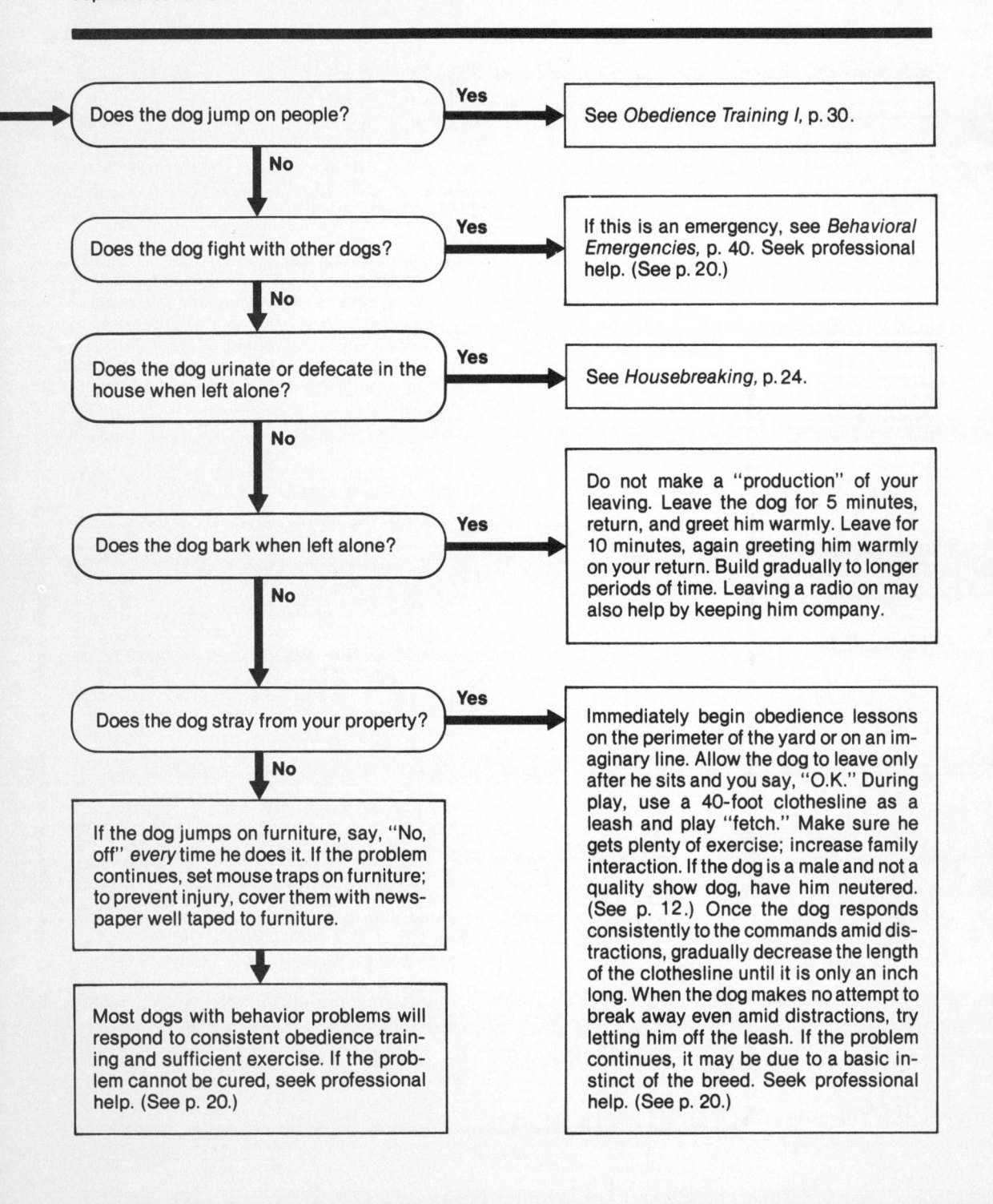

→ Does the dog jump on people? — **Yes** → See *Obedience Training I*, p. 30.

↓ **No**

Does the dog fight with other dogs? — **Yes** → If this is an emergency, see *Behavioral Emergencies*, p. 40. Seek professional help. (See p. 20.)

↓ **No**

Does the dog urinate or defecate in the house when left alone? — **Yes** → See *Housebreaking*, p. 24.

↓ **No**

Does the dog bark when left alone? — **Yes** → Do not make a "production" of your leaving. Leave the dog for 5 minutes, return, and greet him warmly. Leave for 10 minutes, again greeting him warmly on your return. Build gradually to longer periods of time. Leaving a radio on may also help by keeping him company.

↓ **No**

Does the dog stray from your property? — **Yes** → Immediately begin obedience lessons on the perimeter of the yard or on an imaginary line. Allow the dog to leave only after he sits and you say, "O.K." During play, use a 40-foot clothesline as a leash and play "fetch." Make sure he gets plenty of exercise; increase family interaction. If the dog is a male and not a quality show dog, have him neutered. (See p. 12.) Once the dog responds consistently to the commands amid distractions, gradually decrease the length of the clothesline until it is only an inch long. When the dog makes no attempt to break away even amid distractions, try letting him off the leash. If the problem continues, it may be due to a basic instinct of the breed. Seek professional help. (See p. 20.)

↓ **No**

If the dog jumps on furniture, say, "No, off" *every* time he does it. If the problem continues, set mouse traps on furniture; to prevent injury, cover them with newspaper well taped to furniture.

↓

Most dogs with behavior problems will respond to consistent obedience training and sufficient exercise. If the problem cannot be cured, seek professional help. (See p. 20.)

Behavioral Emergencies
(When immediate action is necessary)

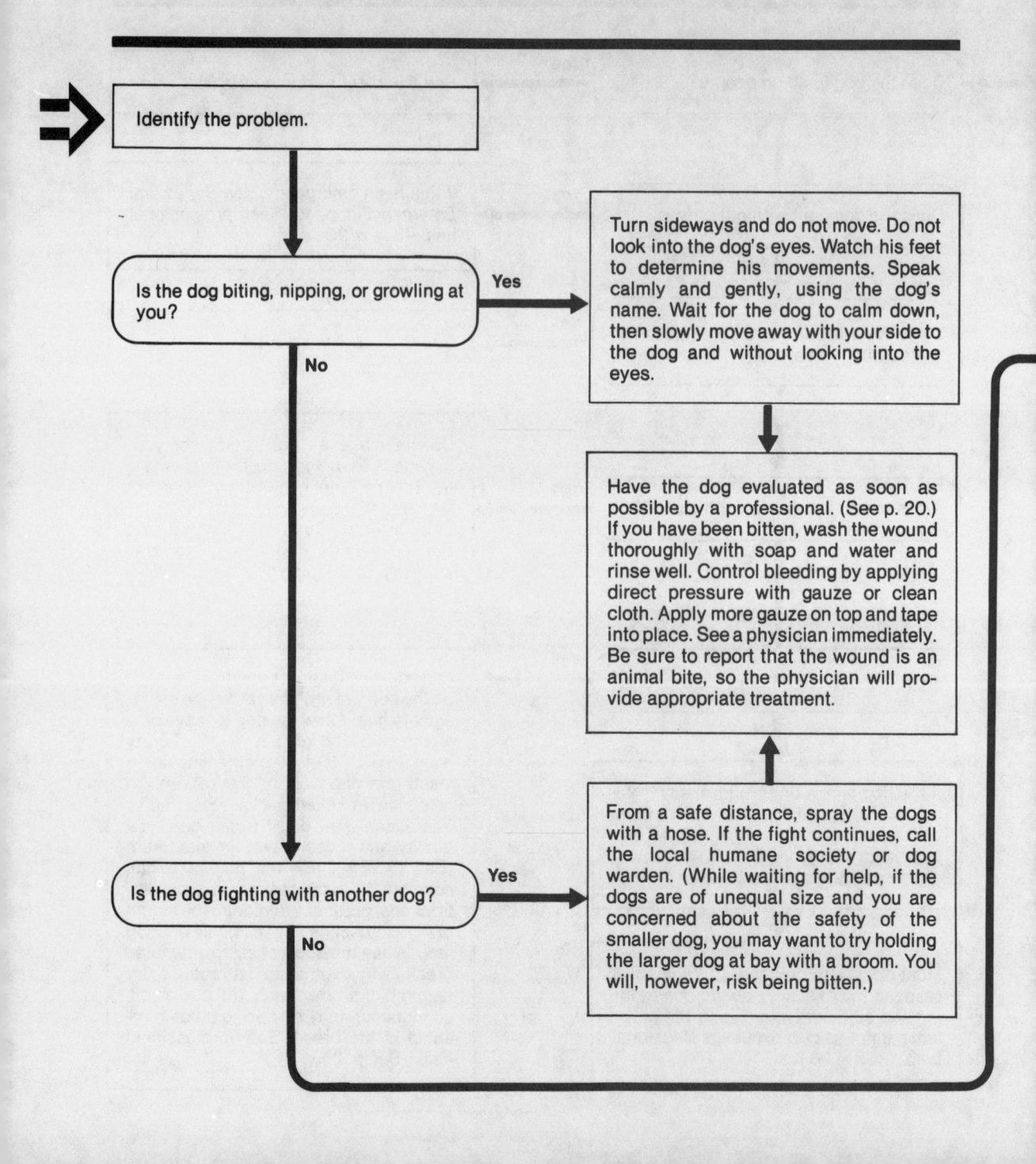

Identify the problem.

Is the dog biting, nipping, or growling at you?

Yes → Turn sideways and do not move. Do not look into the dog's eyes. Watch his feet to determine his movements. Speak calmly and gently, using the dog's name. Wait for the dog to calm down, then slowly move away with your side to the dog and without looking into the eyes.

↓

Have the dog evaluated as soon as possible by a professional. (See p. 20.) If you have been bitten, wash the wound thoroughly with soap and water and rinse well. Control bleeding by applying direct pressure with gauze or clean cloth. Apply more gauze on top and tape into place. See a physician immediately. Be sure to report that the wound is an animal bite, so the physician will provide appropriate treatment.

No ↓

Is the dog fighting with another dog?

Yes → From a safe distance, spray the dogs with a hose. If the fight continues, call the local humane society or dog warden. (While waiting for help, if the dogs are of unequal size and you are concerned about the safety of the smaller dog, you may want to try holding the larger dog at bay with a broom. You will, however, risk being bitten.)

No

If the dog is copulating with another dog, *do not* try to separate them, even if the female is a prize-winning purebred. The dogs are "locked" together and any attempt to separate them could lead to injury. Allow them to complete the act, which may take up to 45 minutes.

If you wish to have the fetuses aborted by a veterinarian, the procedure must be done 1-8 days after conception.

3

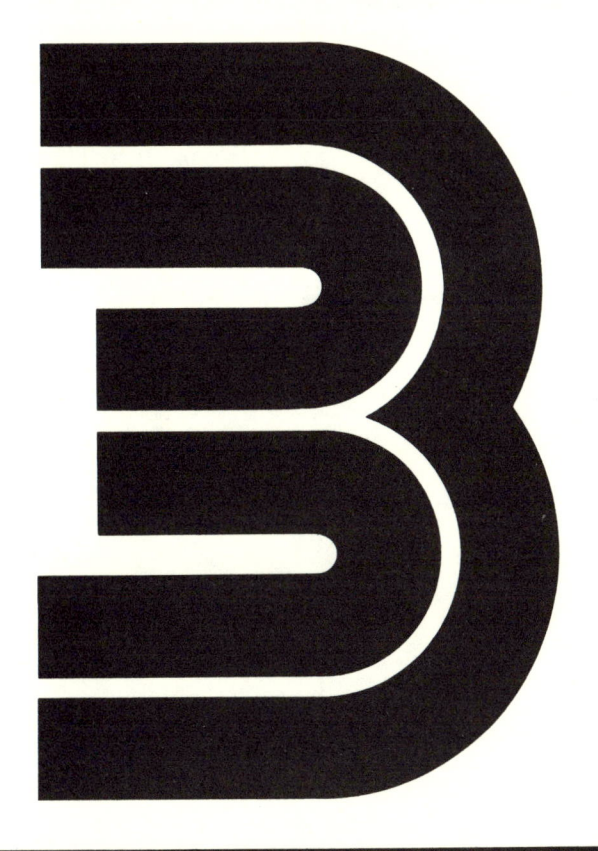

HEALTH PROBLEMS AND EMERGENCY CARE

Strategy Chart: Health Problems & Emergency Care

For proper dog ownership, familiarize yourself with all the precautions and procedures in this section. The chart below outlines some important things to be aware of and their location in this book.

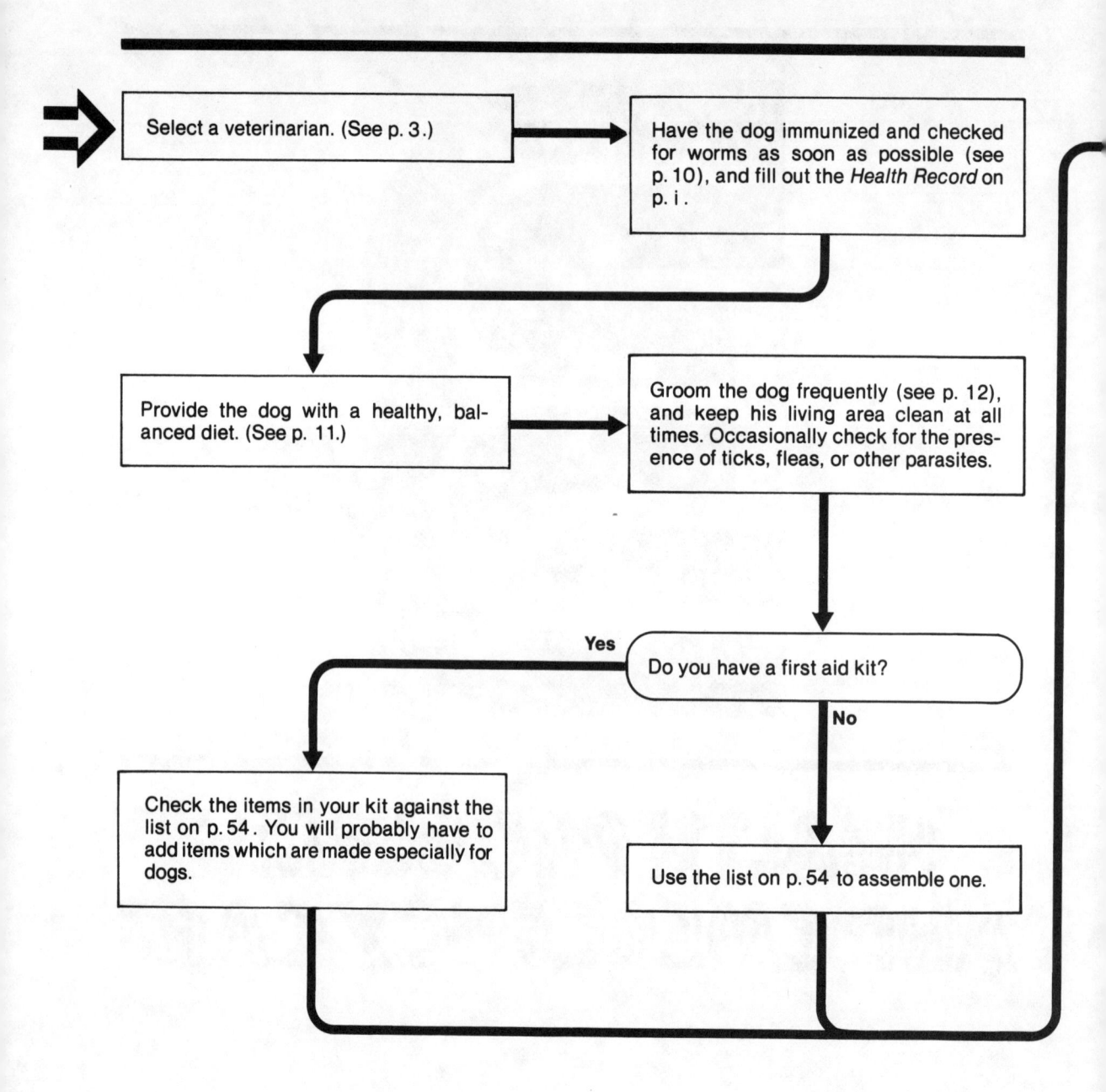

→ Select a veterinarian. (See p. 3.) → Have the dog immunized and checked for worms as soon as possible (see p. 10), and fill out the *Health Record* on p. i.

↓

Provide the dog with a healthy, balanced diet. (See p. 11.) → Groom the dog frequently (see p. 12), and keep his living area clean at all times. Occasionally check for the presence of ticks, fleas, or other parasites.

↓

Do you have a first aid kit?

Yes → Check the items in your kit against the list on p. 54. You will probably have to add items which are made especially for dogs.

No → Use the list on p. 54 to assemble one.

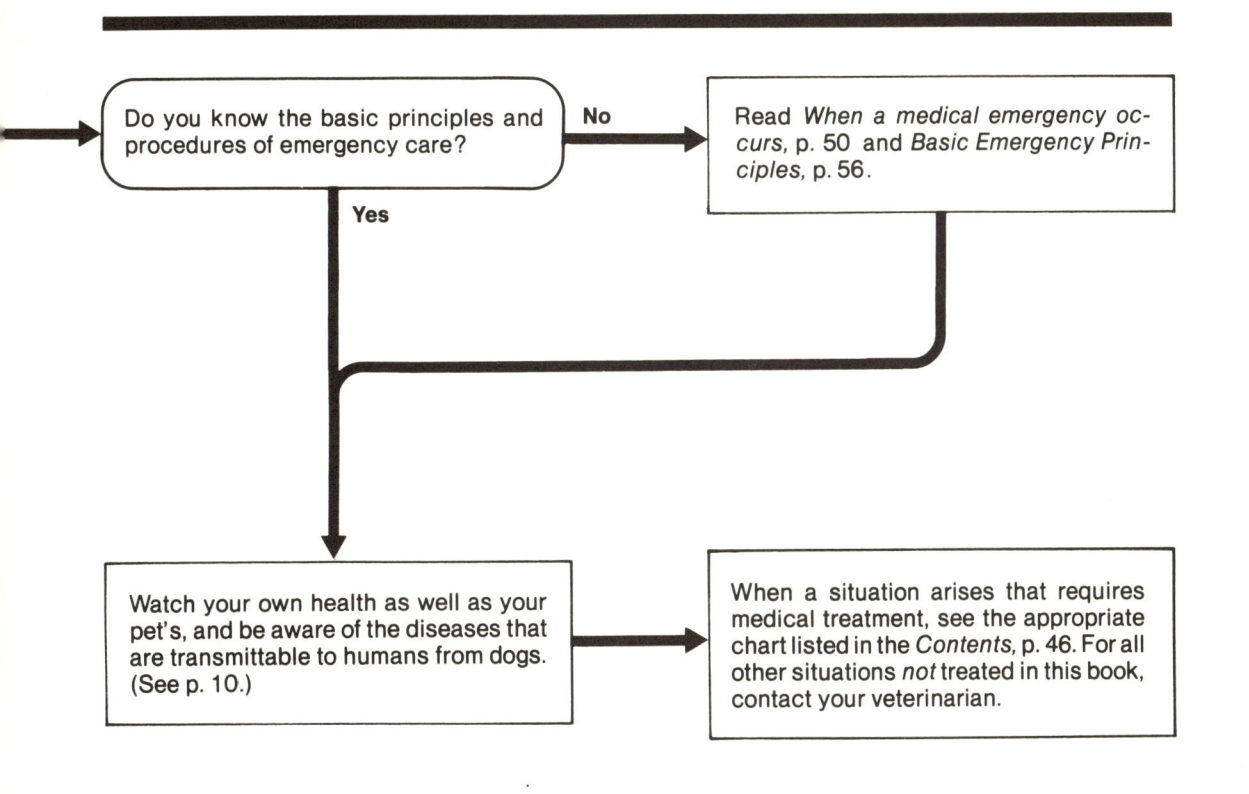

```
┌─────────────────────────┐                    ┌─────────────────────────────────┐
│ Do you know the basic   │       No           │ Read *When a medical emergency  │
│ principles and          │───────────────────▶│ occurs*, p. 50 and *Basic       │
│ procedures of emergency │                    │ Emergency Principles*, p. 56.   │
│ care?                   │                    └─────────────────────────────────┘
└─────────────────────────┘                                    │
         │ Yes                                                 │
         ▼                                                     │
┌─────────────────────────────────┐        ┌──────────────────────────────────┐
│ Watch your own health as well   │        │ When a situation arises that     │
│ as your pet's, and be aware of  │───────▶│ requires medical treatment, see  │
│ the diseases that are           │        │ the appropriate chart listed in  │
│ transmittable to humans from    │        │ the *Contents*, p. 46. For all   │
│ dogs. (See p. 10.)              │        │ other situations *not* treated   │
└─────────────────────────────────┘        │ in this book, contact your       │
                                           │ veterinarian.                    │
                                           └──────────────────────────────────┘
```

Contents:
Health Problems & Emergency Care

Page

Part III: Health Problems & Emergency Care
If there is more than 1 problem, turn to the most serious problem first.

Health Record	i
Introduction	50
Preventing Illness	50
When an Emergency Occurs	50
Taking Your Dog's Temperature	51
Giving Your Dog a Pill	52
Giving Your Dog Liquid Medication	52
Pregnancy	52
Euthanasia	53

	See	
Emergency Principles	Basic Emergency Principles	56
Medical Supplies	Basic Medical Supplies	54
Moving the Seriously Injured Dog	Back & Neck Injuries	78
Moving the Sick or Injured Dog	Transporting to Veterinarian	58
Lifesaving Procedures		
Artificial Respiration	Artificial Respiration & CPR	60
Choking	Choking	62
Drowning	Artificial Respiration & CPR	60
Heart Massage	Artificial Respiration & CPR	60
Illnesses		
Allergic Reaction — drug	Allergic Reaction	76
— food	Allergic Reaction	76
— insect sting	Insect Stings & Bites	88
— pollen	Allergic Reaction	76
Bleeding — anal	Diarrhea, Constipation & Anal Problems	68
— nasal	Nose Problems	92
Breathing Problems — absence of breathing	Artificial Respiration & CPR	60
— choking	Choking	62
— difficult breathing	Breathing Difficulties	64
— rapid breathing	Breathing Difficulties	64
— unconsciousness	Convulsions or Unconsciousness	66
Collapse	Convulsions or Unconsciousness	66

	See	Page
Constipation	Diarrhea, Constipation & Anal Problems	**68**
Convulsions	Convulsions or Unconsciousness	**66**
Diarrhea	Diarrhea, Constipation & Anal Problems	**68**
Epileptic Seizures	Convulsions or Unconsciousness	**66**
Fever	Fever	**70**
Gastrointestinal Problems	Diarrhea, Constipation & Anal Problems	**68**
Nasal Discharge	Nose Problems	**92**
Nosebleed	Nose Problems	**92**
Parasites — internal	Diarrhea, Constipation & Anal Problems	**68**
— external	Insect Stings & Bites	**88**
Sneezing	Nose Problems	**92**
Swelling	Swelling	**98**
Unconsciousness	Convulsions or Unconsciousness	**66**
Vomiting	Vomiting	**72**
Worms	Diarrhea, Constipation & Anal Problems	**68**

Accidents & Injuries

Abdominal Injury	Abdominal & Chest Injuries	**74**
Abrasion	Minor Cuts & Scratches	**82**
Amputation	Puncture & Deep Wounds	**102**
Back Injury	Back & Neck Injuries	**78**
Bleeding — abdominal	Abdominal & Chest Injuries	**74**
— chest	Abdominal & Chest Injuries	**74**
— deep wound	Puncture & Deep Wounds	**102**
— eye	Eye Injuries	**84**
— minor wound	Minor Cuts & Scratches	**82**
— mouth	Tooth & Mouth Injuries	**100**
— nose	Nose Problems	**92**
Burns	Burns	**80**
Chemical Burn — eye	Eye Injuries	**84**
— body	Burns	**80**
Chest Injury	Abdominal & Chest Injuries	**74**
Choking	Choking	**62**
Collapse	Convulsions or Unconsciousness	**66**

continued

Contents (cont.)

	See	**Page**
Convulsions	Convulsions or Unconsciousness	66
Cut — minor	Minor Cuts & Scratches	82
— serious	Puncture & Deep Wounds	102
Drowning	Artificial Respiration & CPR	60
Electric Shock	Burns	80
Eye Injury	Eye Injuries	84
Facial Injury	Head & Facial Injuries	86
Foreign Object — abdomen	Abdominal & Chest Injuries	74
— anus	Diarrhea, Constipation & Anal Problems	68
— chest	Abdominal & Chest Injuries	74
— eye	Eye Injuries	84
— foot	Swelling	98
— mouth	Choking	62
— nose	Nose Problems	92
— throat	Choking	62
Head Injury	Head & Facial Injuries	86
Jaw Injury	Head & Facial Injuries	86
Leg — injury	Leg Fractures, Sprains & Dislocations	90
— wound	Puncture & Deep Wounds	102
Mouth Injury	Tooth & Mouth Injuries	100
Neck Injury	Back & Neck Injuries	78
Nosebleed	Nose Problems	92
Paralysis	Back & Neck Injuries	78
Puncture Wound	Puncture & Deep Wounds	102
Scratch	Minor Cuts & Scratches	82
Smoke Inhalation	Artificial Respiration & CPR	60
Tooth Injury	Tooth & Mouth Injuries	100
Unconsciousness	Convulsions or Unconsciousness	66
Wound — minor	Minor Cuts & Scratches	82
— serious	Puncture & Deep Wounds	102

Poisoning, Bites & Stings

Animal Bites — minor	Minor Cuts & Scratches	82
— serious	Puncture & Deep Wounds	102
Bee Sting	Insect Stings & Bites	88
Chemical Burns	Burns	80
Chemical Poisoning	Poisoning	94

	See	Page
Chiggers	Insect Stings & Bites	**88**
Fleas	Insect Stings & Bites	**88**
Food Poisoning	Poisoning	**94**
Fumes — inhaled	Poisoning	**94**
Insect Sting	Insect Stings & Bites	**88**
Parasites — internal	Diarrhea, Constipation & Anal Problems	**68**
— external	Insect Stings & Bites	**88**
Poisoning — ingested or inhaled	Poisoning	**94**
Scorpion Bite	Insect Stings & Bites	**88**
Snakebite	Snakebite	**96**
Spider Bite	Insect Stings & Bites	**88**
Tick — embedded	Insect Stings & Bites	**88**
Wasp Sting	Insect Stings & Bites	**88**

Exposure to Heat or Cold

Cold Exposure	Cold Exposure & Frostbite	**104**
Frostbite	Cold Exposure & Frostbite	**104**
Heat Exhaustion	Heatstroke & Heat Exhaustion	**106**
Heatstroke	Heatstroke & Heat Exhaustion	**106**
Hypothermia	Cold Exposure & Frostbite	**104**

Part 3
Introduction

These emergency medical procedure charts have been designed to help you handle your dog's potentially dangerous or troublesome illnesses and injuries. The Contents on page 46 will quickly refer you to a specific problem. Restraining the dog is often the first step in giving effective emergency care. Fear and the pain or discomfort of an injury or illness can cause even the most docile dog to bite anyone who causes increased discomfort — even a beloved owner. A list of medical supplies on page 54 will tell you what to have on hand to treat a medical emergency. Many of the supplies will be equally useful in treating your own or your family's medical problems.

The key to good health is preventing illness. Remember to:
— Feed your dog a nutritionally balanced diet. (See p. 11.)
— Give plenty of water.
— Keep the dog and his living area clean at all times.
— Exercise your dog frequently and regularly. The minimum amount of exercise required by a dog is 10-15 minutes of running three times a week. Many breeds require much more. (See p. 4.)
— Be alert to problems. Although a dog cannot speak, he will usually let you know when something is wrong, but often in a subtle way. If you know your dog well and are watching for problems, you will be aware when veterinary assistance is needed.
— Provide care for your dog as soon as you notice a problem. A dog is in many ways more helpless than a child and as much care is necessary. Don't just "wait and see."
— *Never* leave your dog in a hot car. This can lead to heatstroke which can kill some breeds in as little as five minutes.

When a medical emergency occurs:

Remain calm. Take a deep breath, then read these instructions. With all emergencies except when the dog is not breathing (then turn immediately to *Artificial Respiration & CPR,* p. 60), one or two minutes spent getting the situation under control will improve your effectiveness.
Look up the major problem in the *Contents*, p. 46. Before doing anything, read over the chart you'll be using to become familiar with the recommended procedures and equipment.

If a serious emergency occurs that is not listed or if the primary problem is weakness accompanied by pale gums and eyelids, the best procedure is to seek immediate veterinary care; see *Transporting to Veterinarian,* p. 58, before transporting the dog. Evaluation by a veterinarian is necessary if a less serious illness is not listed and there are symptoms such as:
— coughing
— loss of appetite
— stool eating
— problems with bowel or bladder habits
— fatigue
— depression
— excessive thirst
— eye or other discharge without injury
— weight loss.

Provide only emergency care outlined in these charts unless you receive instructions for additional care from a medically trained person by phone or radio.

Use common sense with these charts; only you know your particular situation. The primary rule of emergency care is to cause no further injury.

Most important during any medical emergency — Remember your ABCs:
— Make sure the unconscious dog's *airway* is unobstructed.
— Make sure the dog is *breathing.*
— Be sure the *circulation* of blood is maintained. (Heart is kept pumping, bleeding is controlled, etc.)

Taking Your Dog's Temperature

— Speak gently to the dog.
— Shake down a rectal thermometer. Dip the bulb into petroleum jelly and lubricate up to 1 inch from the bulb.
— Restrain the dog, if necessary: If the dog is not lying down, straddle his back, facing his head. Gently but firmly hold him with your legs, than apply firm, gentle pressure to upper back until he lies down. If there are two persons, the second person can now treat the dog. If you are alone, hold the dog firmly with your legs and one arm, or strap with ties, belts, etc., before treating.
— With one hand, grasp the dog's tail. With the other, gently ease the thermometer about 1 inch into the dog's anus, rotating it slowly back and forth.
— After three minutes, remove the thermometer and hold the bulb with a piece of tissue to read the temperature. Wash the thermometer with soap and lukewarm water.
— See appropriate chart for treatment.

Giving Your Dog a Pill

Never give a pill to a dog that is unconscious or having breathing difficulty. Speak gently to the dog. Have the dog sit with his head raised slightly upward. Use one of the following methods:
— Wrap the pill in pieces of food, such as meat or cheese, or surround the pill with a glob of peanut butter. First give some non-medicated food to the dog, then give the medicated piece or hunk of peanut butter.
— Smear butter on the pill to lubricate it. Place your left hand (or, if you are left-handed, your right hand) over the dog's muzzle. Gently squeeze his upper lips up and out of the way. With your fingers on his gums, tilt his muzzle slightly upward. Holding the pill between the thumb and forefinger of your other hand, place the pill on the back of the throat. Rub his throat or tap his nose to encourage swallowing. If the dog licks his nose, he has probably swallowed the pill.

Giving Your Dog Liquid Medication

Put the appropriate amount of medication into a plastic container or device such as a bulb baster, syringe with no needle, or narrow-necked bottle. Toward the back of the mouth, pull one of the lower lips away from the teeth. Slowly pour or push the medication into the area. Allow the dog time to swallow. When all medication has been given, rub the throat to assure swallowing. If the dog licks his nose, he has probably swallowed the medication.

Pregnancy

If you suspect your dog has become pregnant either by your design or by chance, make an appointment with your veterinarian. He will be able to confirm the pregnancy, discuss with you what you need to know for each step of the pregnancy, in case problems should occur, and tell you what materials you should have on hand.

If your dog is birthing and is straining to expel a puppy, you may help by pulling the partially exposed part of the puppy gently out of the vagina with a soft towel or cloth; when the mother stops to take a rest, firmly hold the puppy still, and begin pulling again when her efforts resume.

If a puppy appears not to be breathing, wipe away any membrane gently from the face and head with a soft cloth, and quickly rub him briskly in a towel. If there is still no response, see *Artificial Respiration & CPR,* p. 60.

For all other problems with the mother or her puppies, contact a veterinarian.

Euthanasia

At some point in your relationship with your dog, it may be necessary to make the decision of whether to put him to sleep. The decision is a moral and a medical one and should be made only after extensive thought. All too frequently, an owner has second thoughts about his decision.

If you are considering putting to sleep a vicious dog, first try to have the problem cured by a professional dog trainer (see p. 20) and/or try to have the dog placed in another home where his temperament will not be a problem before putting the dog to sleep.

If your dog is very sick or in great pain, discuss your options with your veterinarian. If possible, do not make a hasty decision. If you have *any* questions, ask; the veterinarian will understand your concern. Do not hesitate to obtain a second opinion for any reason; a reputable veterinarian, like a reputable physician, will not object to your desire for a second opinion in this situation or in any other involving a major medical decision.

Basic Medical Supplies

Basic Medical Supplies for use with *Your Dog: An Owner's Manual*

The supplies specified are divided into two lists: medical supplies, which should be kept separate for emergency care and first aid, and basic supplies, which may be used for other purposes as well as for emergencies. The designated provisions include only those supplies required in these charts. Most of these items are available in supermarkets or pharmacies.

Medical Supplies
activated charcoal tablets (medicinal)
adhesive tape
antibiotic ointment (Neosporin, Bacitracin, etc.)
antidiarrheal (Kaopectate, Pepto-Bismol, etc.)
antihistamine (Chlor-Trimeton, Contac, Dristan, etc.)
cotton
flea spray, powder, or dip
lip balm (ChapStick, etc.)
mineral oil
needle-nosed pliers or forceps
non-adhering sterile gauze
petroleum jelly
rectal thermometer
rubbing alcohol
snakebite kit*
sterile gauze bandages (1", 2")
sterile gauze pads
syringe (with no needle)
syrup of ipecac
tick spray, powder, or dip
tweezers

*If in a region populated by poisonous snakes.

Basic Supplies that can be used as medical supplies
aluminum foil
baking soda
blankets
clean cloth (sheeting, etc.)
egg whites
handkerchiefs
ice
knife
matches
measuring spoons
mild soap (Ivory, etc.)
milk
plastic bags or wrap
razor blade
rubber gloves
scissors
tissue
tomato juice
towels
vegetable oil

Basic Emergency Principles

The primary rule of emergency care is: Cause no further injury.

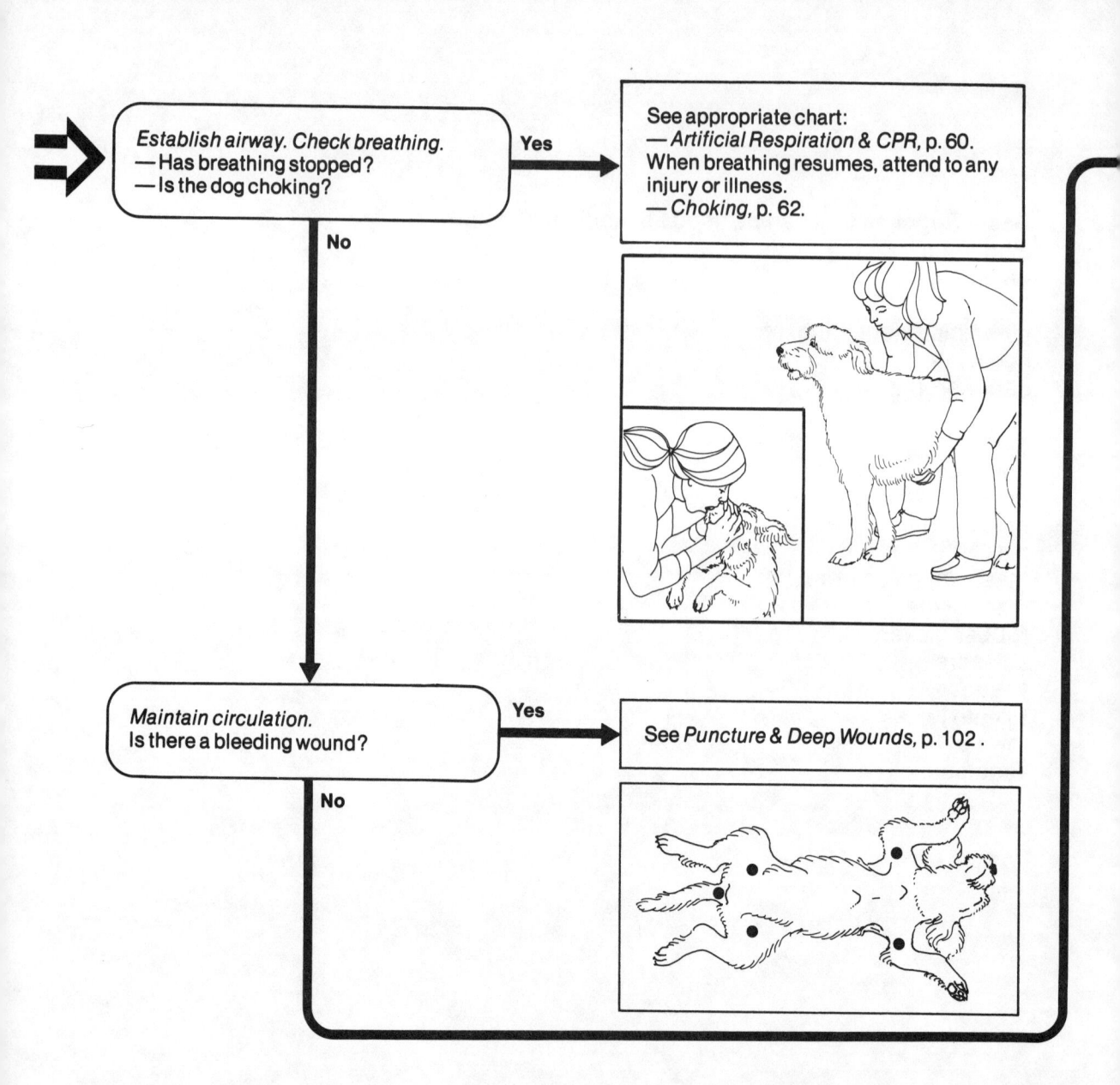

Establish airway. Check breathing.
— Has breathing stopped?
— Is the dog choking?

Yes → See appropriate chart:
— *Artificial Respiration & CPR*, p. 60.
When breathing resumes, attend to any injury or illness.
— *Choking*, p. 62.

No ↓

Maintain circulation.
Is there a bleeding wound?

Yes → See *Puncture & Deep Wounds*, p. 102.

No ↓

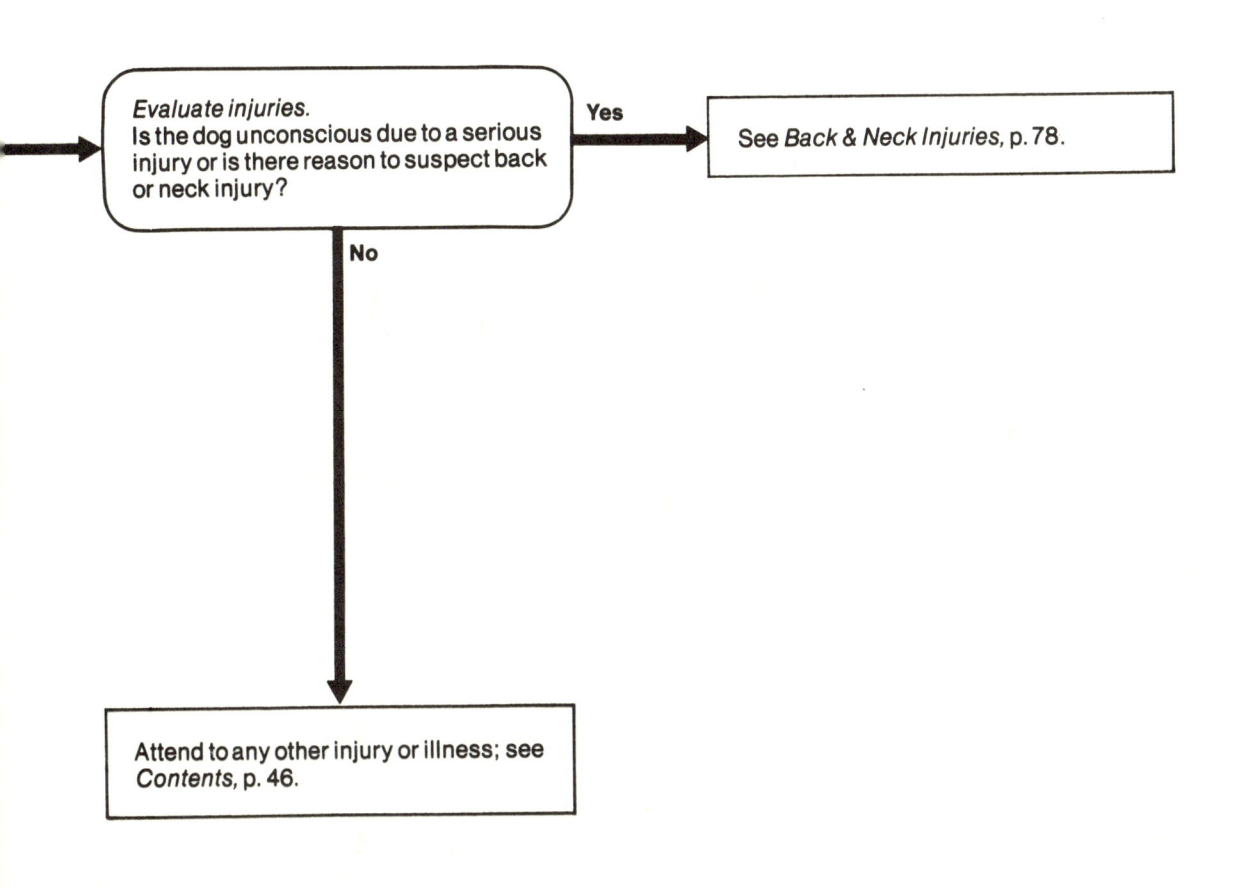

Evaluate injuries.
Is the dog unconscious due to a serious injury or is there reason to suspect back or neck injury? — **Yes** → See *Back & Neck Injuries,* p. 78.

No

Attend to any other injury or illness; see *Contents,* p. 46.

Transporting to Veterinarian

Attend to any injury, illness, etc. (see *Contents*, p. 46), before proceeding through this chart.

Restrain the dog, if necessary, and have him lie quietly. (See Restraining Procedure box.)

Restraining Procedure:
Muzzling:* For a short-nosed dog, wrap a thick towel firmly around head and neck, securing ends. For a long-nosed dog, bring a long gauze or cloth strip under chin; make a single half-knot on top, bring back under chin, tie a single half-knot again, and bring ends behind head, tying securely with a bow. Do not knot.
Restraining: If the dog is not lying down, straddle his back, facing his head. Gently but firmly hold him with your legs. To have him sit, press on hind quarters; to have him lie, apply firm, gentle pressure gradually to upper back.

Has breathing stopped?

Yes → See *Artificial Respiration & CPR,* p. 60. When breathing resumes, return to this chart.

No →

Obtain a blanket, board, ironing board, door, mattress board, etc., or, for a small dog, a box or other carrier.

*Do not muzzle, or if muzzled, remove immediately, if the dog is unconscious, convulsing, vomiting, having difficulty breathing, or there is blood or other matter in mouth.

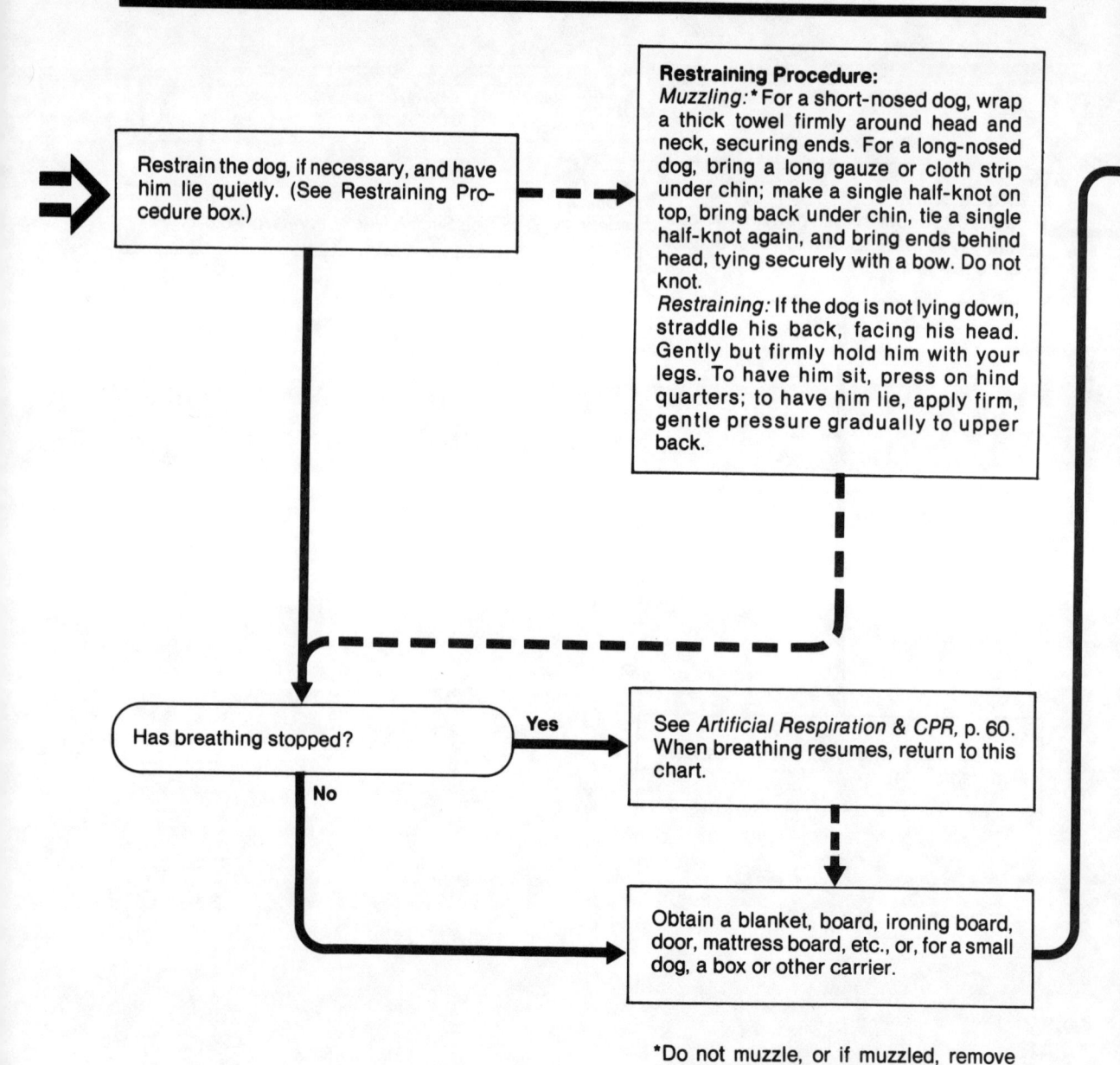

To transport a dog with back, neck, head, leg, abdomen, chest, or serious eye or facial injuries, see *Back & Neck Injuries*, p. 78.

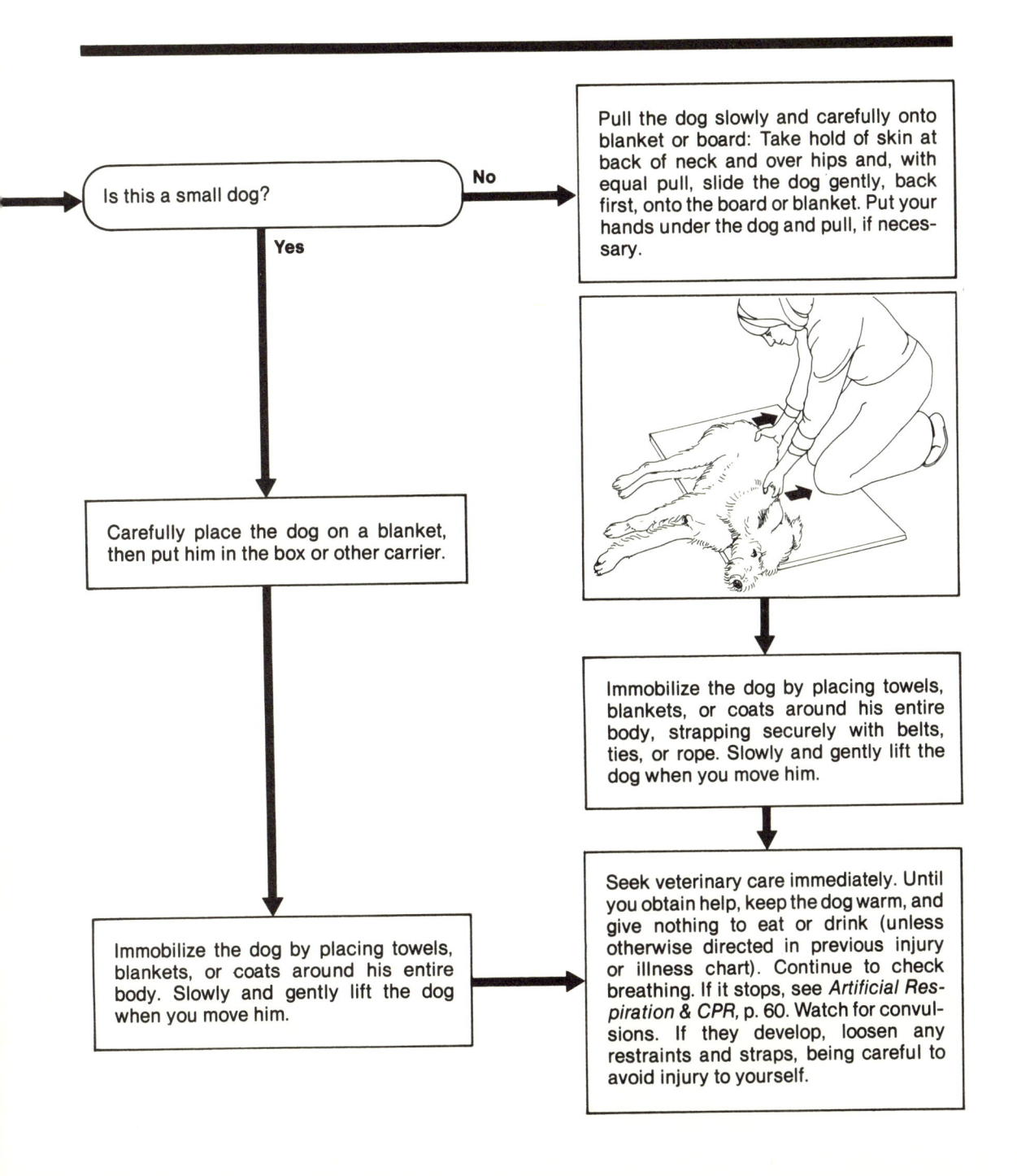

Calm the dog by speaking gently.

Is this a small dog?

No → Pull the dog slowly and carefully onto blanket or board: Take hold of skin at back of neck and over hips and, with equal pull, slide the dog gently, back first, onto the board or blanket. Put your hands under the dog and pull, if necessary.

Yes ↓

Carefully place the dog on a blanket, then put him in the box or other carrier.

↓

Immobilize the dog by placing towels, blankets, or coats around his entire body. Slowly and gently lift the dog when you move him.

↓

Immobilize the dog by placing towels, blankets, or coats around his entire body, strapping securely with belts, ties, or rope. Slowly and gently lift the dog when you move him.

↓

Seek veterinary care immediately. Until you obtain help, keep the dog warm, and give nothing to eat or drink (unless otherwise directed in previous injury or illness chart). Continue to check breathing. If it stops, see *Artificial Respiration & CPR*, p. 60. Watch for convulsions. If they develop, loosen any restraints and straps, being careful to avoid injury to yourself.

Artificial Respiration & CPR

For a newborn puppy, rub briskly in a towel. If still no breathing, see chart below.

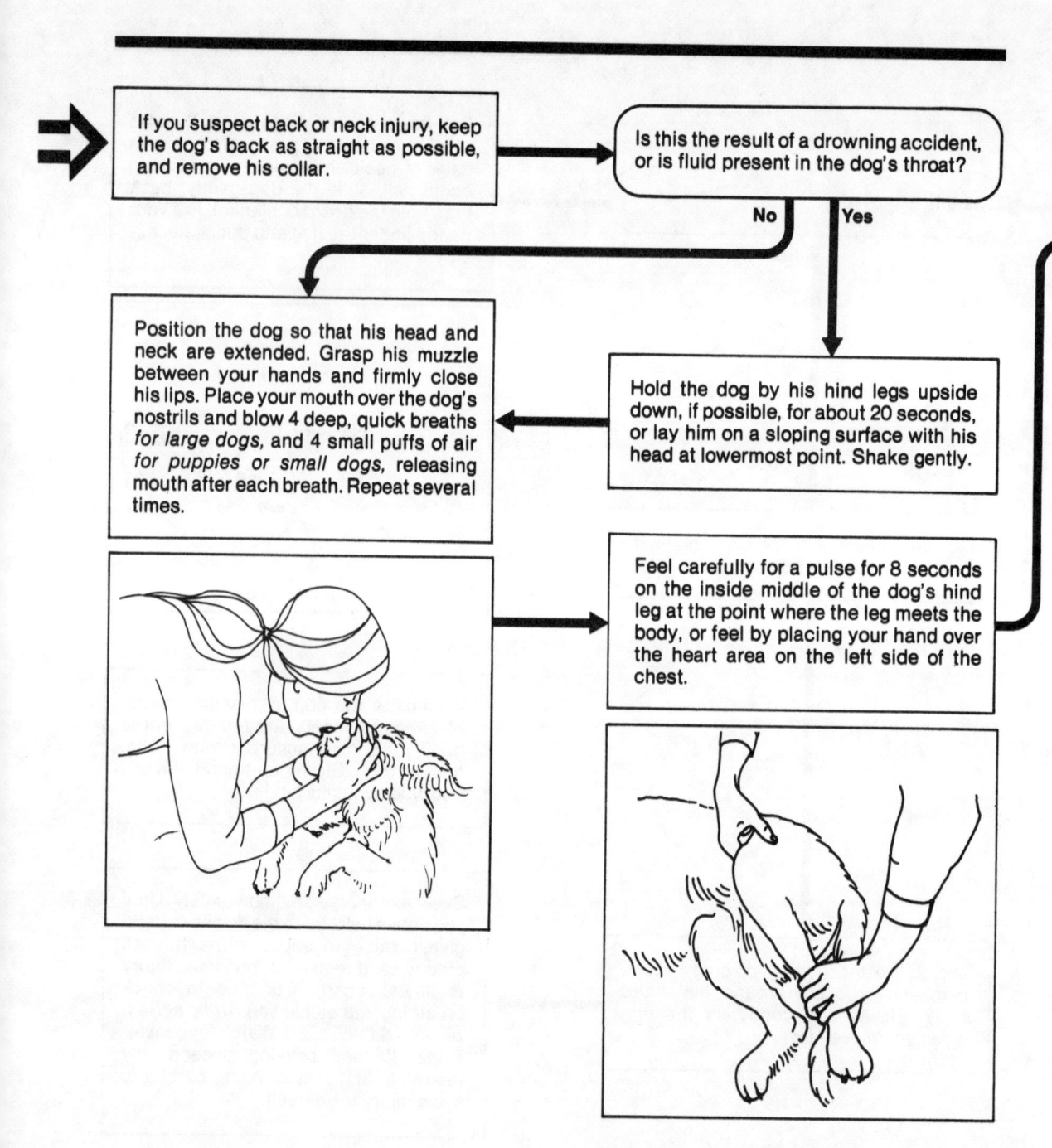

➡️ If you suspect back or neck injury, keep the dog's back as straight as possible, and remove his collar.

Is this the result of a drowning accident, or is fluid present in the dog's throat?

No / **Yes**

Position the dog so that his head and neck are extended. Grasp his muzzle between your hands and firmly close his lips. Place your mouth over the dog's nostrils and blow 4 deep, quick breaths *for large dogs,* and 4 small puffs of air *for puppies or small dogs,* releasing mouth after each breath. Repeat several times.

Hold the dog by his hind legs upside down, if possible, for about 20 seconds, or lay him on a sloping surface with his head at lowermost point. Shake gently.

Feel carefully for a pulse for 8 seconds on the inside middle of the dog's hind leg at the point where the leg meets the body, or feel by placing your hand over the heart area on the left side of the chest.

If the dog was eating, and/or you suspect obstruction of the throat by a foreign object, see *Choking,* **p. 62. If in an area where smoke or noxious fumes are present, move the dog into fresh air.**

This chart should only be used if breathing has stopped. Check for breathing by shaking the dog gently, shouting his name, tickling his nostrils with a weed, tissue, or feather, and/or holding a mirror or piece of glass to his nostrils. (Condensation means the dog is breathing.)

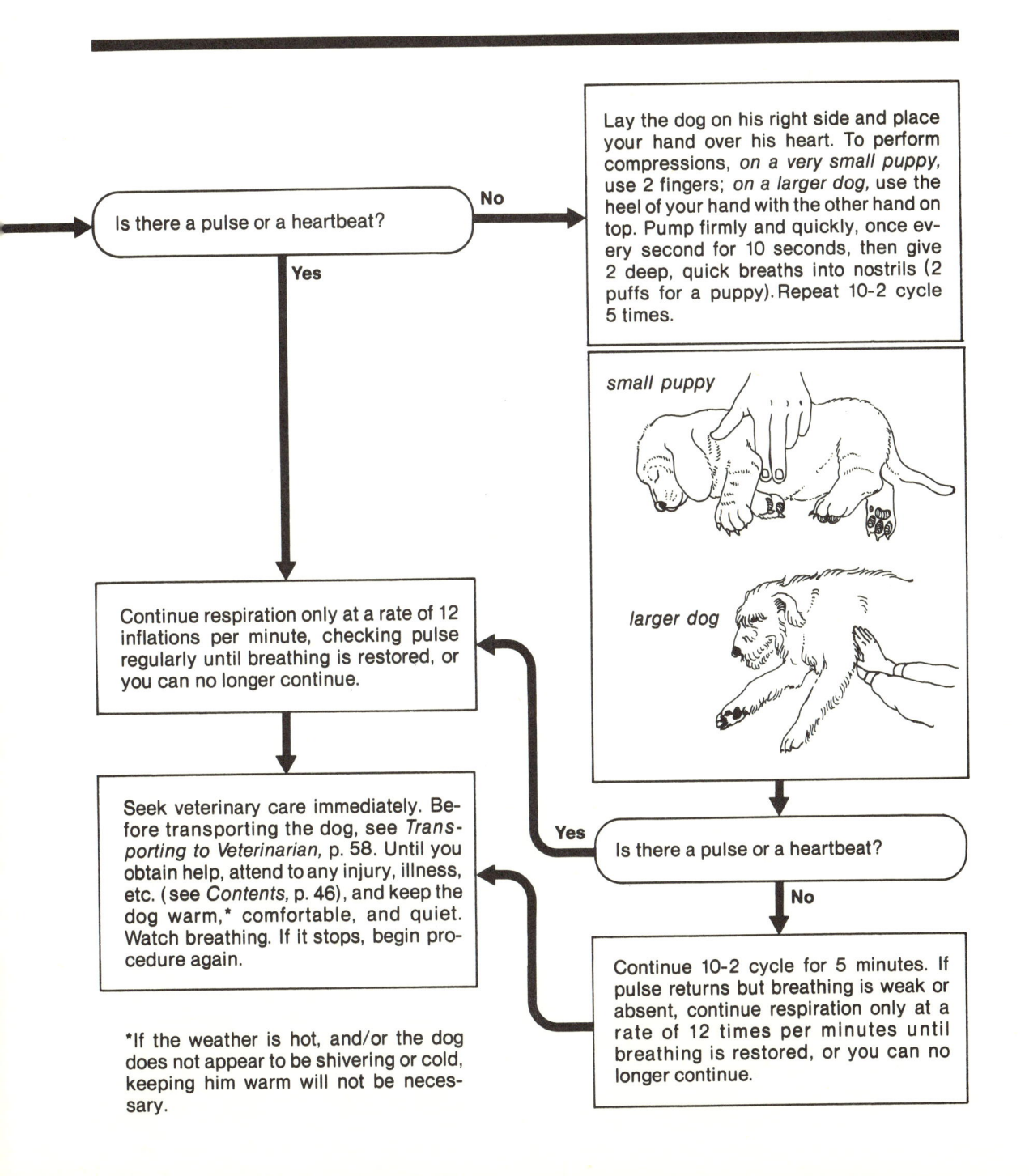

Is there a pulse or a heartbeat?

No → Lay the dog on his right side and place your hand over his heart. To perform compressions, *on a very small puppy,* use 2 fingers; *on a larger dog,* use the heel of your hand with the other hand on top. Pump firmly and quickly, once every second for 10 seconds, then give 2 deep, quick breaths into nostrils (2 puffs for a puppy). Repeat 10-2 cycle 5 times.

small puppy

larger dog

Yes ↓

Continue respiration only at a rate of 12 inflations per minute, checking pulse regularly until breathing is restored, or you can no longer continue.

Seek veterinary care immediately. Before transporting the dog, see *Transporting to Veterinarian,* p. 58. Until you obtain help, attend to any injury, illness, etc. (see *Contents,* p. 46), and keep the dog warm,* comfortable, and quiet. Watch breathing. If it stops, begin procedure again.

*If the weather is hot, and/or the dog does not appear to be shivering or cold, keeping him warm will not be necessary.

Yes ← Is there a pulse or a heartbeat?

No ↓

Continue 10-2 cycle for 5 minutes. If pulse returns but breathing is weak or absent, continue respiration only at a rate of 12 times per minutes until breathing is restored, or you can no longer continue.

Choking

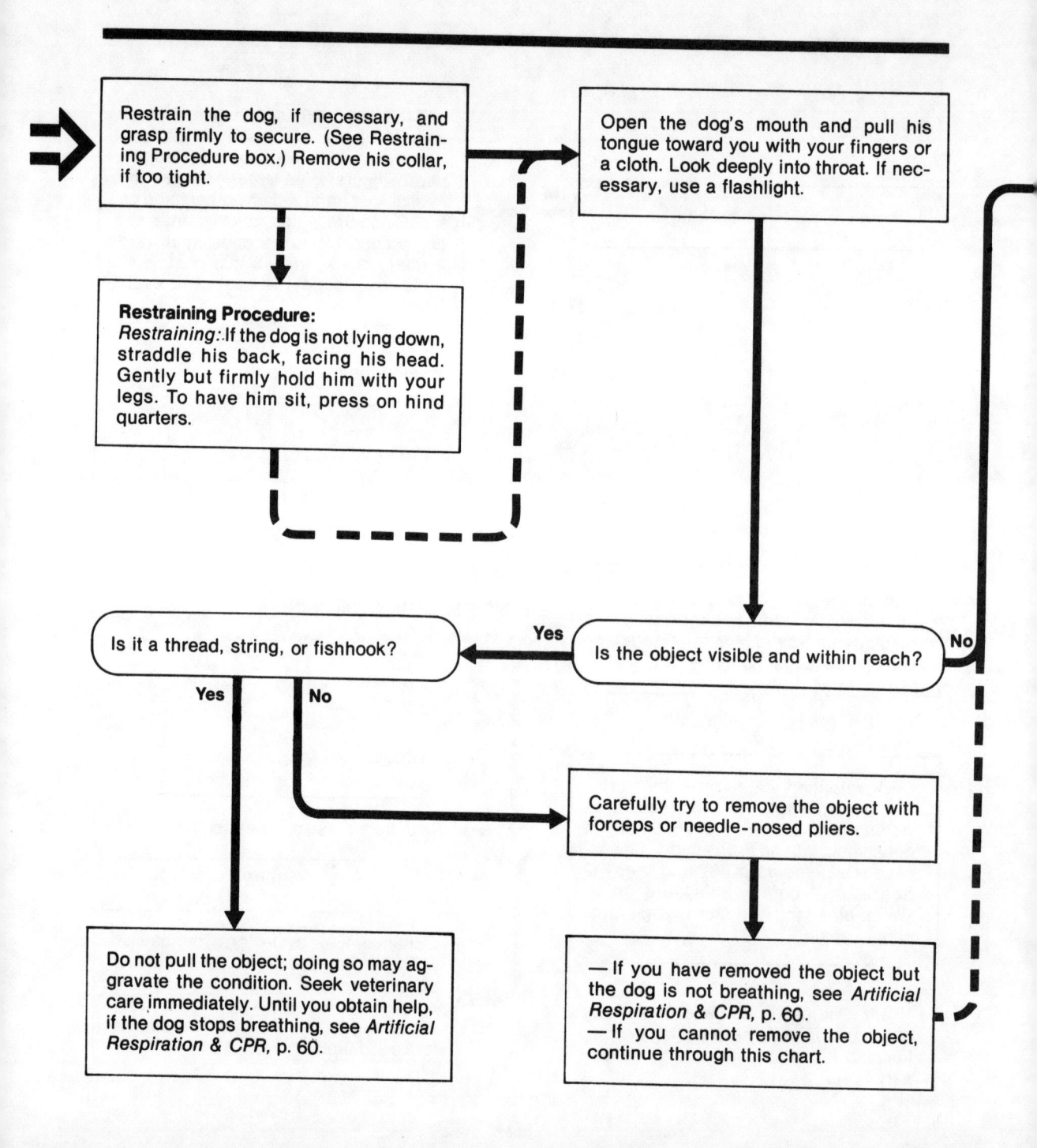

Do not use this chart if the dog is able to cough.

→ Restrain the dog, if necessary, and grasp firmly to secure. (See Restraining Procedure box.) Remove his collar, if too tight.

Restraining Procedure:
Restraining: If the dog is not lying down, straddle his back, facing his head. Gently but firmly hold him with your legs. To have him sit, press on hind quarters.

Open the dog's mouth and pull his tongue toward you with your fingers or a cloth. Look deeply into throat. If necessary, use a flashlight.

Is the object visible and within reach?

Yes → Is it a thread, string, or fishhook?

- **Yes:** Do not pull the object; doing so may aggravate the condition. Seek veterinary care immediately. Until you obtain help, if the dog stops breathing, see *Artificial Respiration & CPR*, p. 60.

- **No:** Carefully try to remove the object with forceps or needle-nosed pliers.
  — If you have removed the object but the dog is not breathing, see *Artificial Respiration & CPR*, p. 60.
  — If you cannot remove the object, continue through this chart.

No →

Possible Signs & Symptoms: *obvious foreign object in throat/difficult breathing/heavy drooling/gagging/violent pawing at face/blue tongue or mouth/extreme anxiety or agitation/sudden loss of consciousness.*

Similar symptoms may indicate a circulatory or respiratory problem. If the dog wasn't eating and you do not suspect choking, see *Breathing Difficulties*, p. 64.

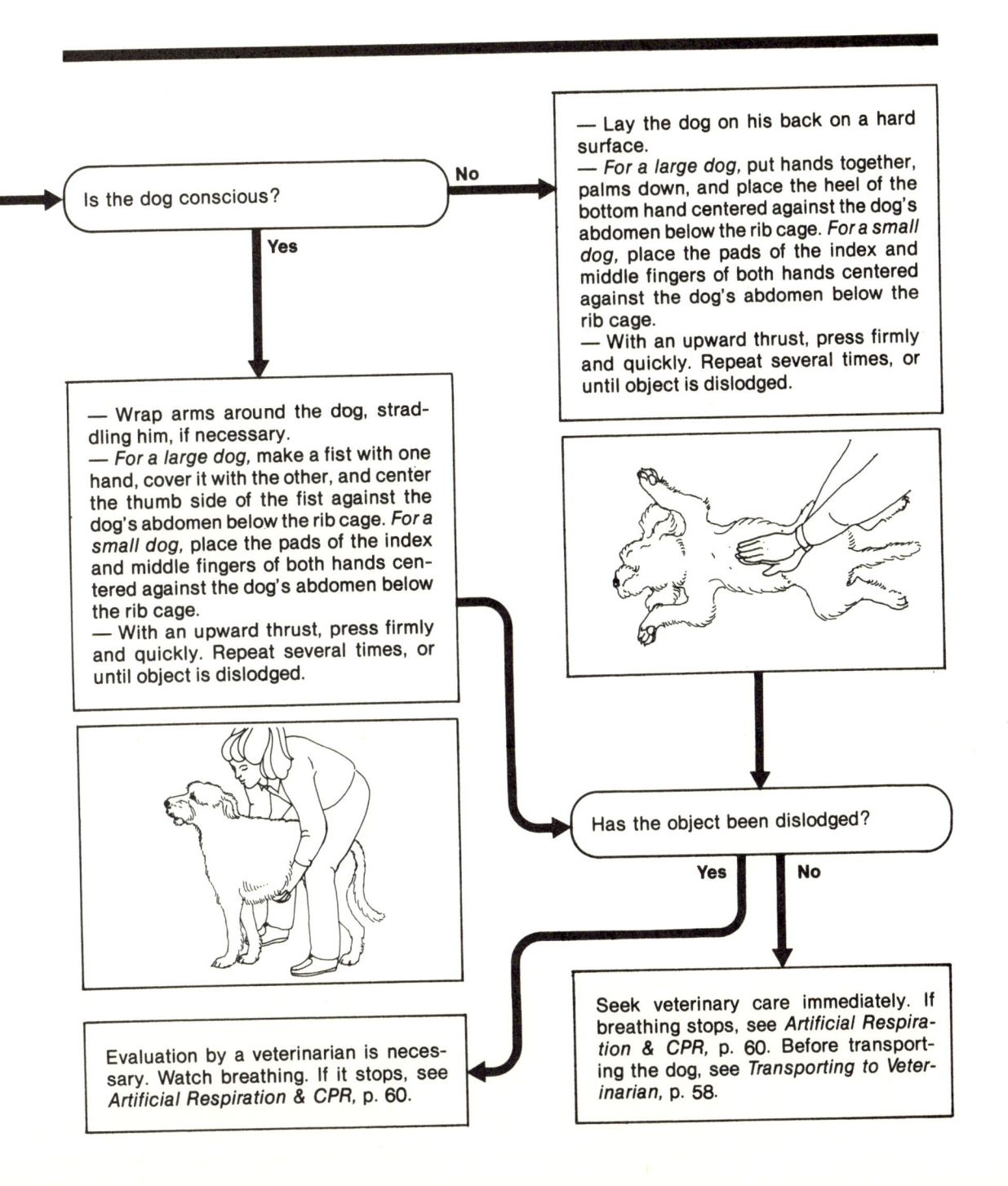

Calm the dog by speaking gently.

Is the dog conscious?

No
— Lay the dog on his back on a hard surface.
— *For a large dog,* put hands together, palms down, and place the heel of the bottom hand centered against the dog's abdomen below the rib cage. *For a small dog,* place the pads of the index and middle fingers of both hands centered against the dog's abdomen below the rib cage.
— With an upward thrust, press firmly and quickly. Repeat several times, or until object is dislodged.

Yes
— Wrap arms around the dog, straddling him, if necessary.
— *For a large dog,* make a fist with one hand, cover it with the other, and center the thumb side of the fist against the dog's abdomen below the rib cage. *For a small dog,* place the pads of the index and middle fingers of both hands centered against the dog's abdomen below the rib cage.
— With an upward thrust, press firmly and quickly. Repeat several times, or until object is dislodged.

Has the object been dislodged?

Yes
Evaluation by a veterinarian is necessary. Watch breathing. If it stops, see *Artificial Respiration & CPR*, p. 60.

No
Seek veterinary care immediately. If breathing stops, see *Artificial Respiration & CPR*, p. 60. Before transporting the dog, see *Transporting to Veterinarian*, p. 58.

Breathing Difficulties

If the dog was eating and is choking, see *Choking,* p. 62. If breathing has stopped, see *Artificial Respiration & CPR,* p. 60.

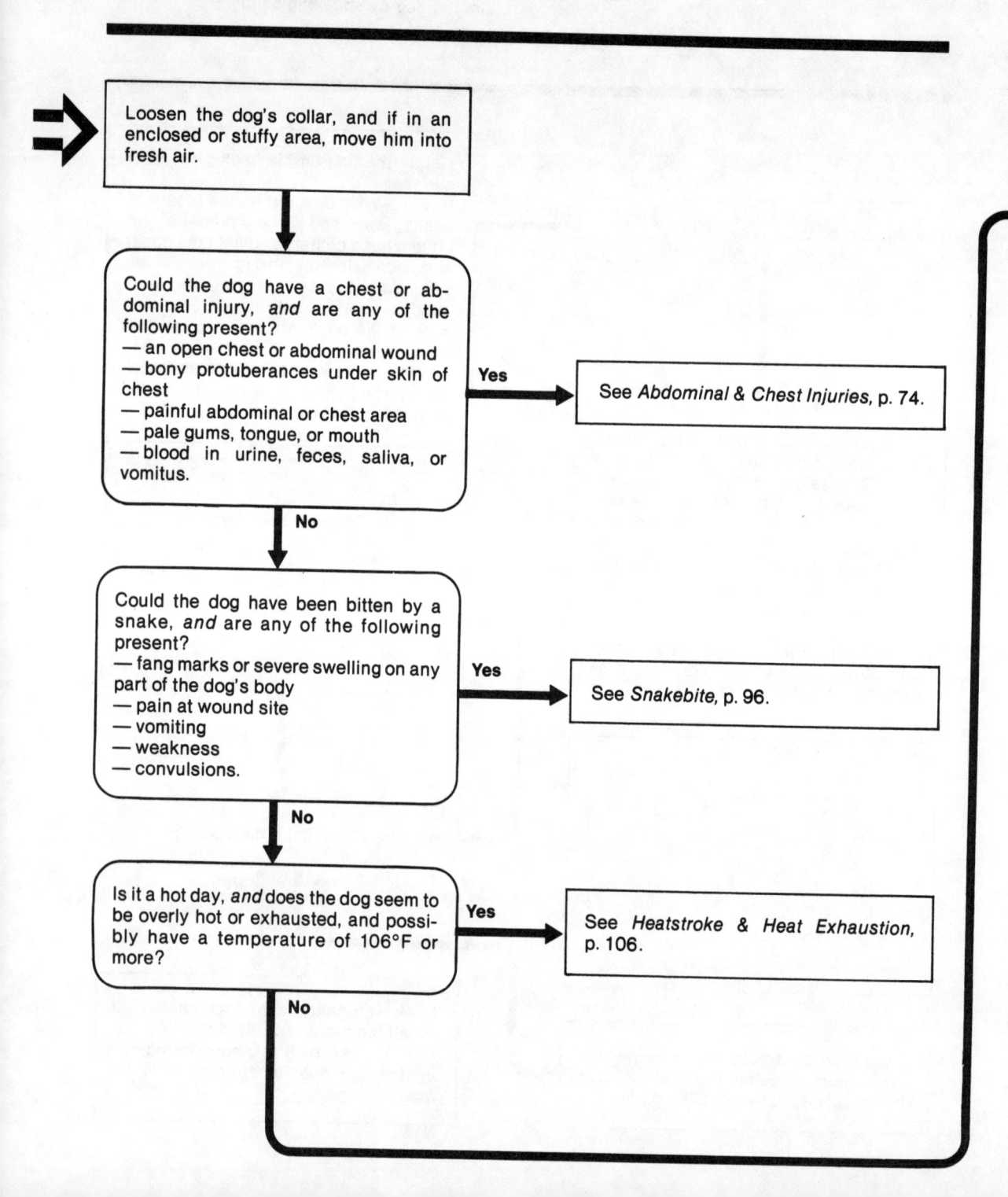

→ Loosen the dog's collar, and if in an enclosed or stuffy area, move him into fresh air.

↓

Could the dog have a chest or abdominal injury, *and* are any of the following present?
— an open chest or abdominal wound
— bony protuberances under skin of chest
— painful abdominal or chest area
— pale gums, tongue, or mouth
— blood in urine, feces, saliva, or vomitus.

Yes → See *Abdominal & Chest Injuries,* p. 74.

No ↓

Could the dog have been bitten by a snake, *and* are any of the following present?
— fang marks or severe swelling on any part of the dog's body
— pain at wound site
— vomiting
— weakness
— convulsions.

Yes → See *Snakebite,* p. 96.

No ↓

Is it a hot day, *and* does the dog seem to be overly hot or exhausted, and possibly have a temperature of 106°F or more?

Yes → See *Heatstroke & Heat Exhaustion,* p. 106.

No ↓

Possible Signs & Symptoms: *deep, shallow, rapid, or irregular breathing/gasping/blueness of lips, tongue, gums or inner eyelids/staring/ loss of consciousness.*

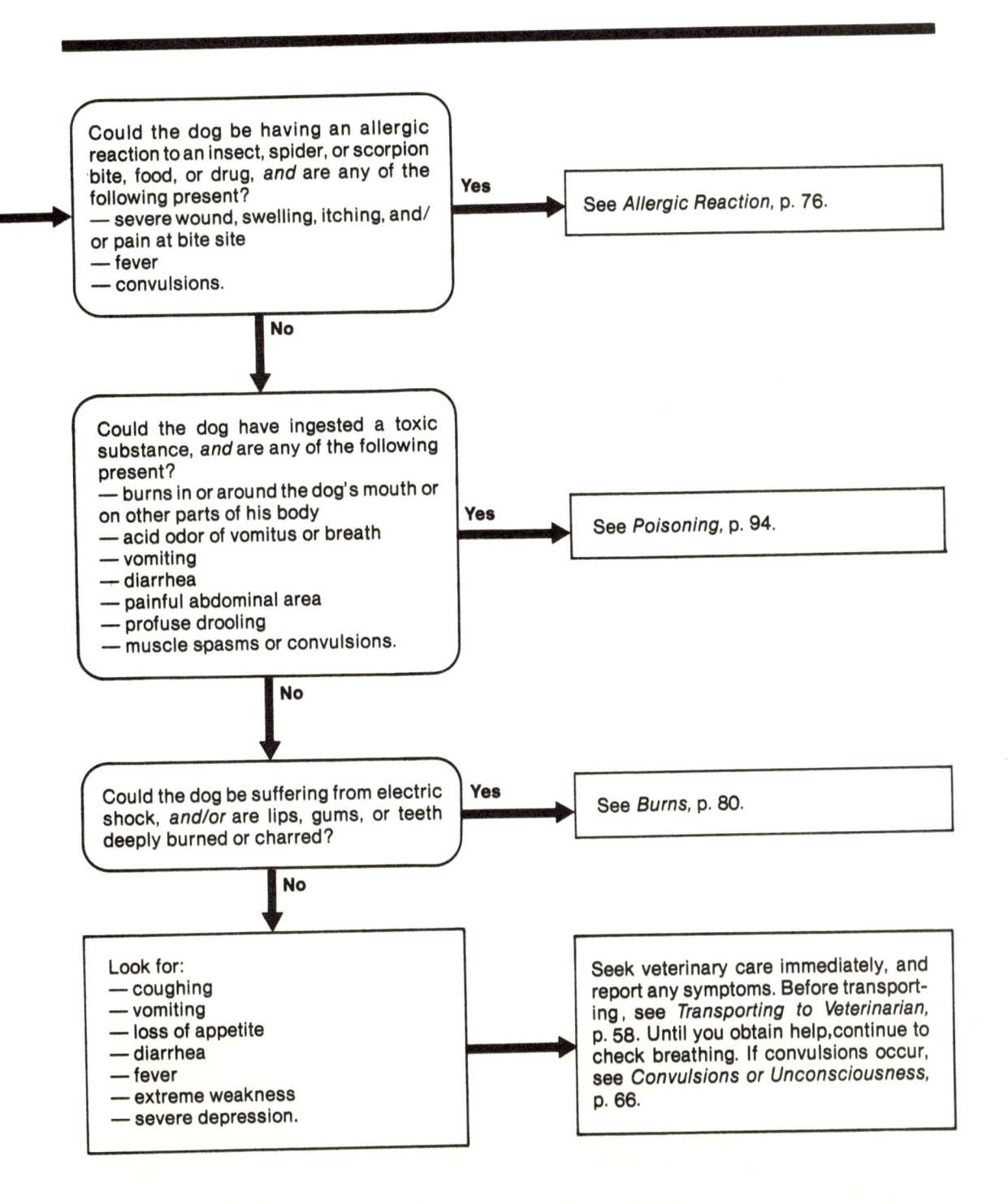

Calm the dog by speaking gently.

Could the dog be having an allergic reaction to an insect, spider, or scorpion bite, food, or drug, *and* are any of the following present?
— severe wound, swelling, itching, and/or pain at bite site
— fever
— convulsions.

Yes → See *Allergic Reaction*, p. 76.

No ↓

Could the dog have ingested a toxic substance, *and* are any of the following present?
— burns in or around the dog's mouth or on other parts of his body
— acid odor of vomitus or breath
— vomiting
— diarrhea
— painful abdominal area
— profuse drooling
— muscle spasms or convulsions.

Yes → See *Poisoning*, p. 94.

No ↓

Could the dog be suffering from electric shock, *and/or* are lips, gums, or teeth deeply burned or charred?

Yes → See *Burns*, p. 80.

No ↓

Look for:
— coughing
— vomiting
— loss of appetite
— diarrhea
— fever
— extreme weakness
— severe depression.

→ Seek veterinary care immediately, and report any symptoms. Before transporting, see *Transporting to Veterinarian*, p. 58. Until you obtain help, continue to check breathing. If convulsions occur, see *Convulsions or Unconsciousness*, p. 66.

Convulsions or Unconsciousness

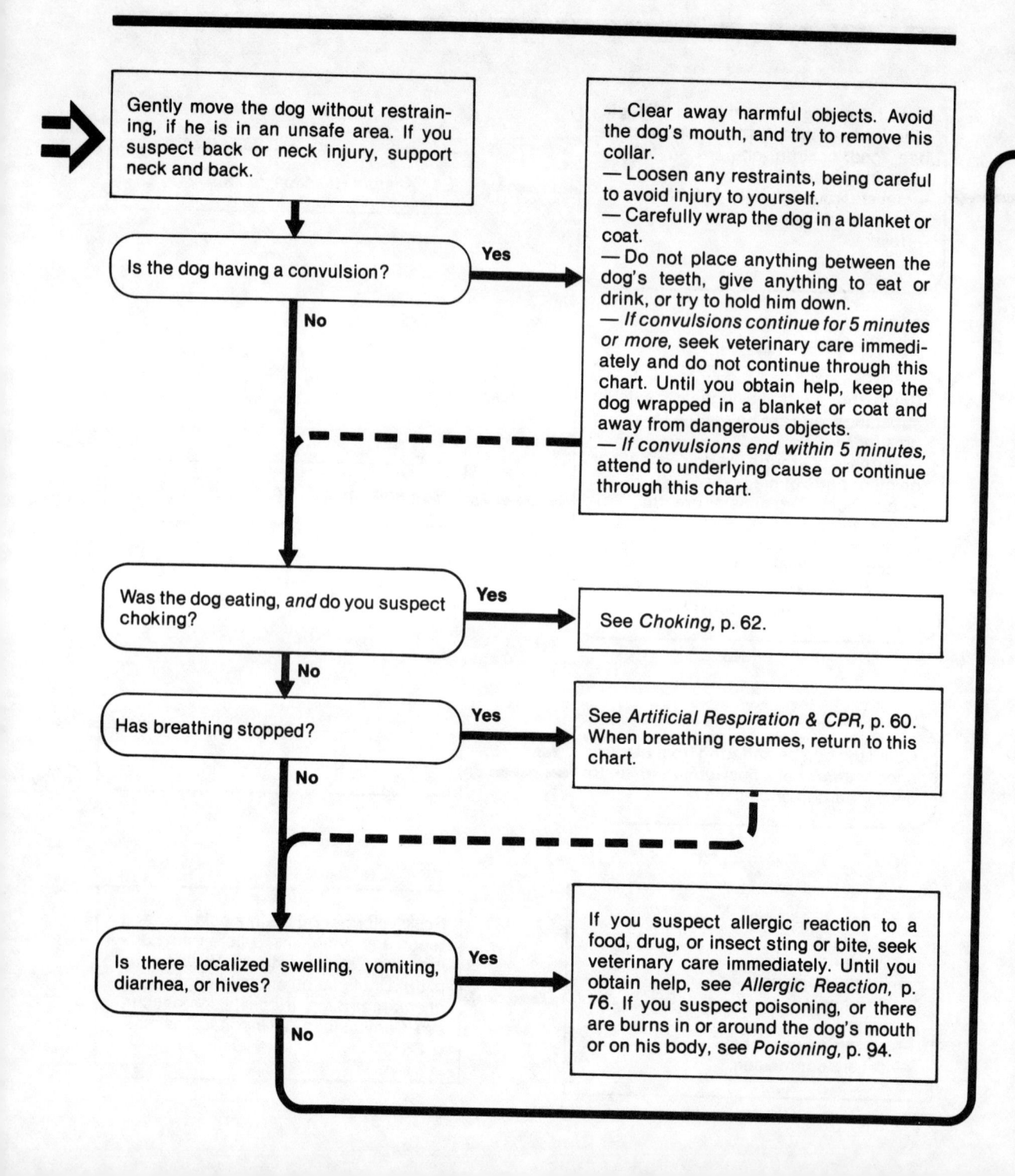

→ Gently move the dog without restraining, if he is in an unsafe area. If you suspect back or neck injury, support neck and back.

↓

Is the dog having a convulsion? — Yes →
- Clear away harmful objects. Avoid the dog's mouth, and try to remove his collar.
- Loosen any restraints, being careful to avoid injury to yourself.
- Carefully wrap the dog in a blanket or coat.
- Do not place anything between the dog's teeth, give anything to eat or drink, or try to hold him down.
- *If convulsions continue for 5 minutes or more,* seek veterinary care immediately and do not continue through this chart. Until you obtain help, keep the dog wrapped in a blanket or coat and away from dangerous objects.
- *If convulsions end within 5 minutes,* attend to underlying cause or continue through this chart.

No ↓

Was the dog eating, *and* do you suspect choking? — Yes → See *Choking*, p. 62.

No ↓

Has breathing stopped? — Yes → See *Artificial Respiration & CPR*, p. 60. When breathing resumes, return to this chart.

No ↓

Is there localized swelling, vomiting, diarrhea, or hives? — Yes → If you suspect allergic reaction to a food, drug, or insect sting or bite, seek veterinary care immediately. Until you obtain help, see *Allergic Reaction*, p. 76. If you suspect poisoning, or there are burns in or around the dog's mouth or on his body, see *Poisoning*, p. 94.

No ↓

Possible Signs & Symptoms: *involuntary jerking of muscles/loss of bowel and bladder control/stiffening of body/loss of consciousness.*

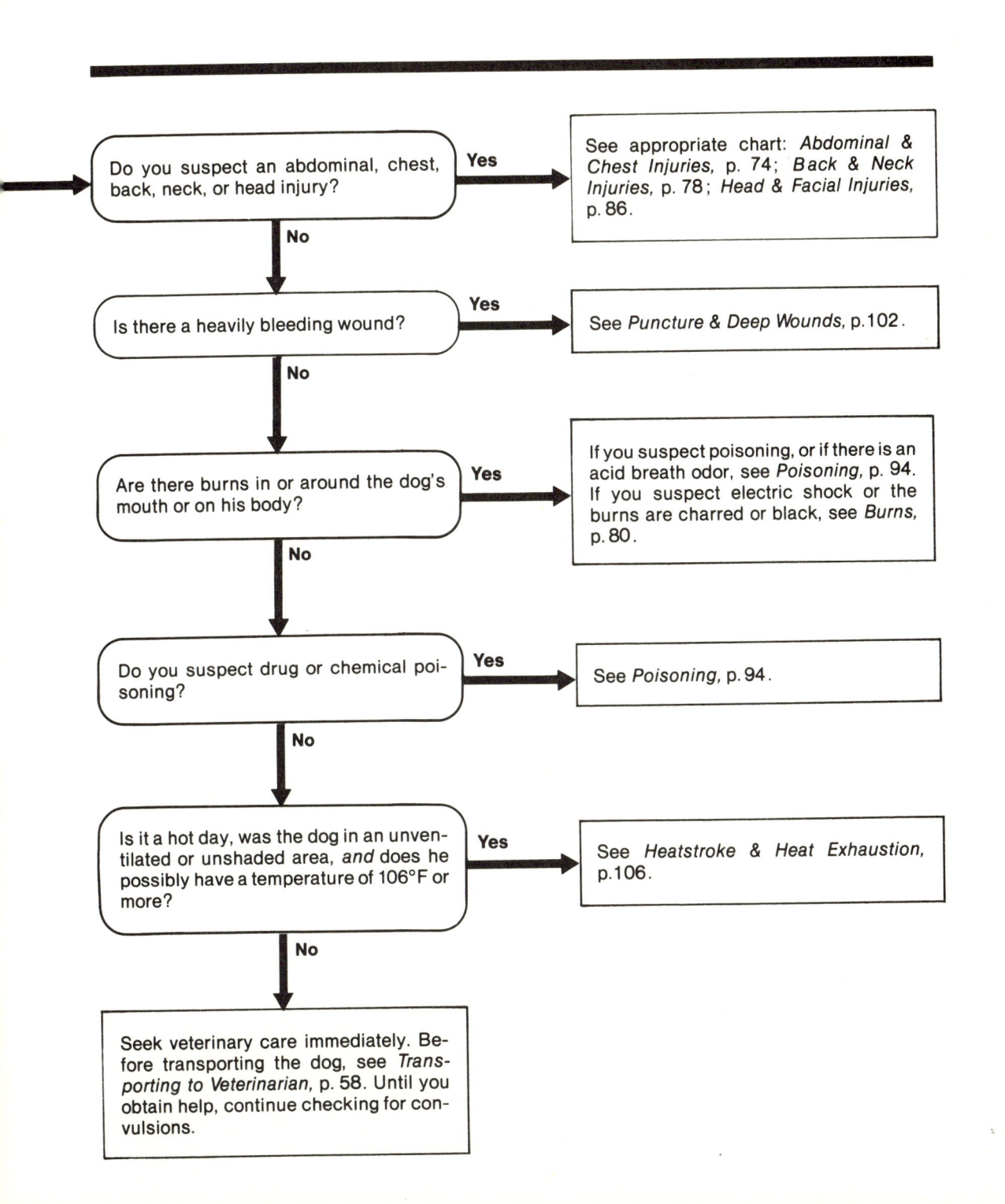

- Do you suspect an abdominal, chest, back, neck, or head injury? → **Yes** → See appropriate chart: *Abdominal & Chest Injuries*, p. 74; *Back & Neck Injuries*, p. 78; *Head & Facial Injuries*, p. 86.
- **No** ↓
- Is there a heavily bleeding wound? → **Yes** → See *Puncture & Deep Wounds*, p. 102.
- **No** ↓
- Are there burns in or around the dog's mouth or on his body? → **Yes** → If you suspect poisoning, or if there is an acid breath odor, see *Poisoning*, p. 94. If you suspect electric shock or the burns are charred or black, see *Burns*, p. 80.
- **No** ↓
- Do you suspect drug or chemical poisoning? → **Yes** → See *Poisoning*, p. 94.
- **No** ↓
- Is it a hot day, was the dog in an unventilated or unshaded area, *and* does he possibly have a temperature of 106°F or more? → **Yes** → See *Heatstroke & Heat Exhaustion*, p. 106.
- **No** ↓
- Seek veterinary care immediately. Before transporting the dog, see *Transporting to Veterinarian*, p. 58. Until you obtain help, continue checking for convulsions.

Diarrhea, Constipation & Anal Problems
(Including Worms & Foreign Object)

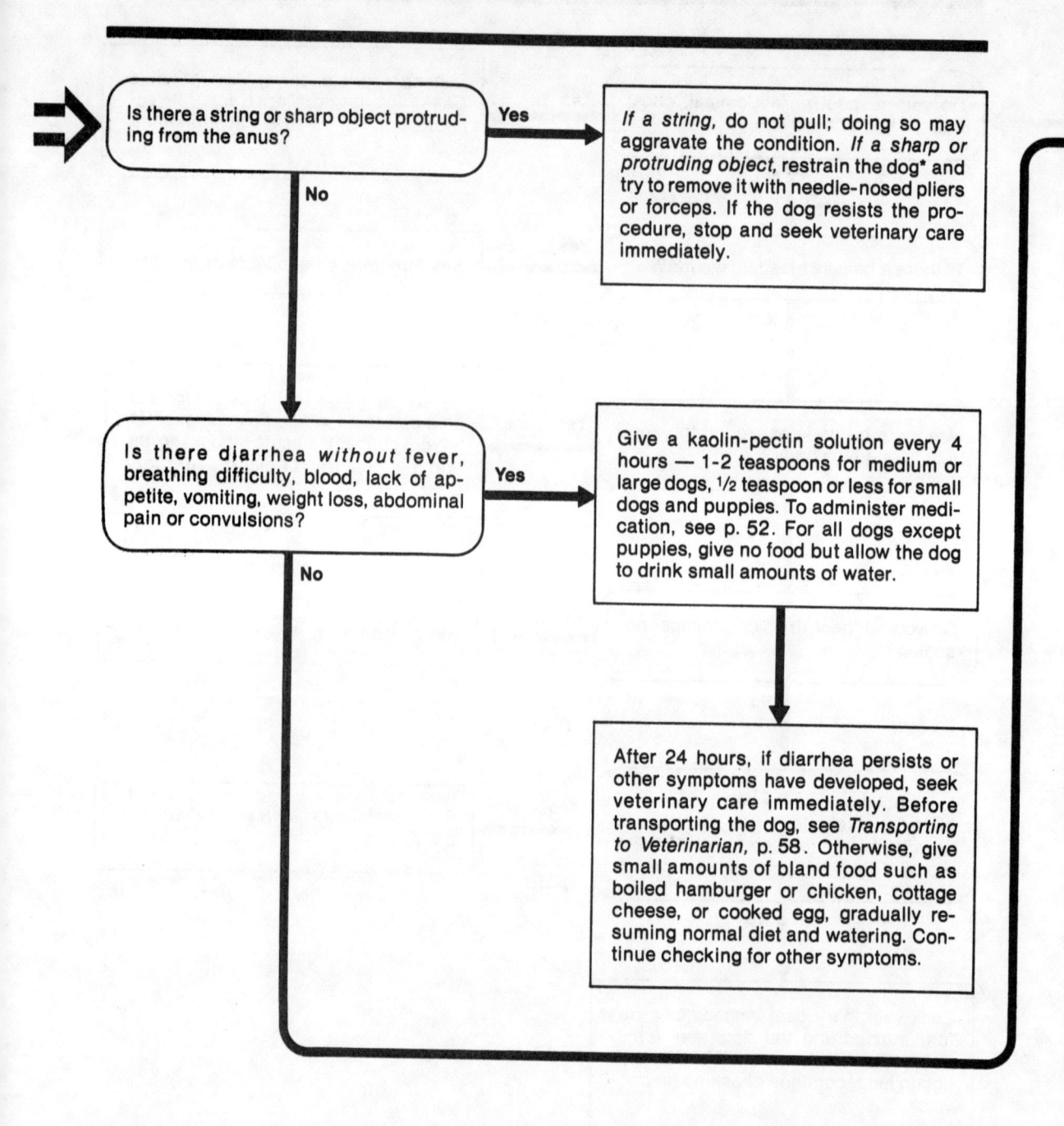

➡️ **Is there a string or sharp object protruding from the anus?** — **Yes** → *If a string,* do not pull; doing so may aggravate the condition. *If a sharp or protruding object,* restrain the dog* and try to remove it with needle-nosed pliers or forceps. If the dog resists the procedure, stop and seek veterinary care immediately.

↓ **No**

Is there diarrhea *without* fever, breathing difficulty, blood, lack of appetite, vomiting, weight loss, abdominal pain or convulsions? — **Yes** → Give a kaolin-pectin solution every 4 hours — 1-2 teaspoons for medium or large dogs, 1/2 teaspoon or less for small dogs and puppies. To administer medication, see p. 52. For all dogs except puppies, give no food but allow the dog to drink small amounts of water.

↓

After 24 hours, if diarrhea persists or other symptoms have developed, seek veterinary care immediately. Before transporting the dog, see *Transporting to Veterinarian,* p. 58. Otherwise, give small amounts of bland food such as boiled hamburger or chicken, cottage cheese, or cooked egg, gradually resuming normal diet and watering. Continue checking for other symptoms.

↓ **No**

If the dog may have ingested a poison, see *Poisoning*, **p. 94.**

Possible Signs & Symptoms: *diarrhea/constipation/sharp object or string protruding from the anus/blood or white worm-like objects in stool/rubbing, scratching, or licking anal area.*

Calm the dog by speaking gently.

Is there constipation or strained passage of feces, or is the anus blocked? — **Yes** →

— Check anal area. If hair is matted over the anus, restrain the dog* and carefully clip the hair away. Gently wash the area and apply petroleum jelly to any irritation.
— If constipation continues, and listlessness and/or lack of appetite develop, mix mineral oil (1/2 teaspoon or less for small dogs and puppies, 1-2 teaspoons for medium or large dogs) well into the dog's food once a day, or add water to dry food.
— If constipation or straining persists after 1 day, seek veterinary care immediately.

No ↓

Look for:
— swelling, lumps, or red masses around anal area
— swollen and/or painful abdominal area
— bloody or tar-like stools
— white worm-like objects in stool
— changes in the dog's coat
— loss of weight or appetite
— coughing and/or sneezing
— vomiting
— fever
— breathing difficulty
— weakness or depression
— frequent urination.

Seek veterinary care immediately and report any symptoms. If there are bloody or tar-like stools, extreme weakness, or other serious symptoms, see *Transporting to Veterinarian*, p. 58, before transporting the dog. Until you obtain help, if the dog is sneezing or coughing, keep him warm. If he vomits, do not give food or water, but allow him to lick ice cubes. Watch for convulsions. If these occur, see *Convulsions or Unconsciousness*, p. 66.

* Restraining Procedure:
Muzzling: Do not muzzle, or if muzzled, remove immediately, if the dog is unconscious, convulsing, vomiting, having difficulty breathing, or there is blood or other matter in mouth. For a short-nosed dog, wrap a thick towel firmly around head and neck, securing ends. For a long-nosed dog, bring a long gauze or cloth strip under chin; make a single half-knot on top, bring back under chin, tie a single half-knot again, and bring ends behind head, tying securely with a bow. Do not knot.
Restraining: If the dog is not lying down, straddle his back, facing his head. Gently but firmly hold him with your legs.
— If there are two persons, second person can now treat the dog.
— If you are alone, hold the dog firmly with your legs and one arm, or strap with ties, belts, etc., before treating.

Fever

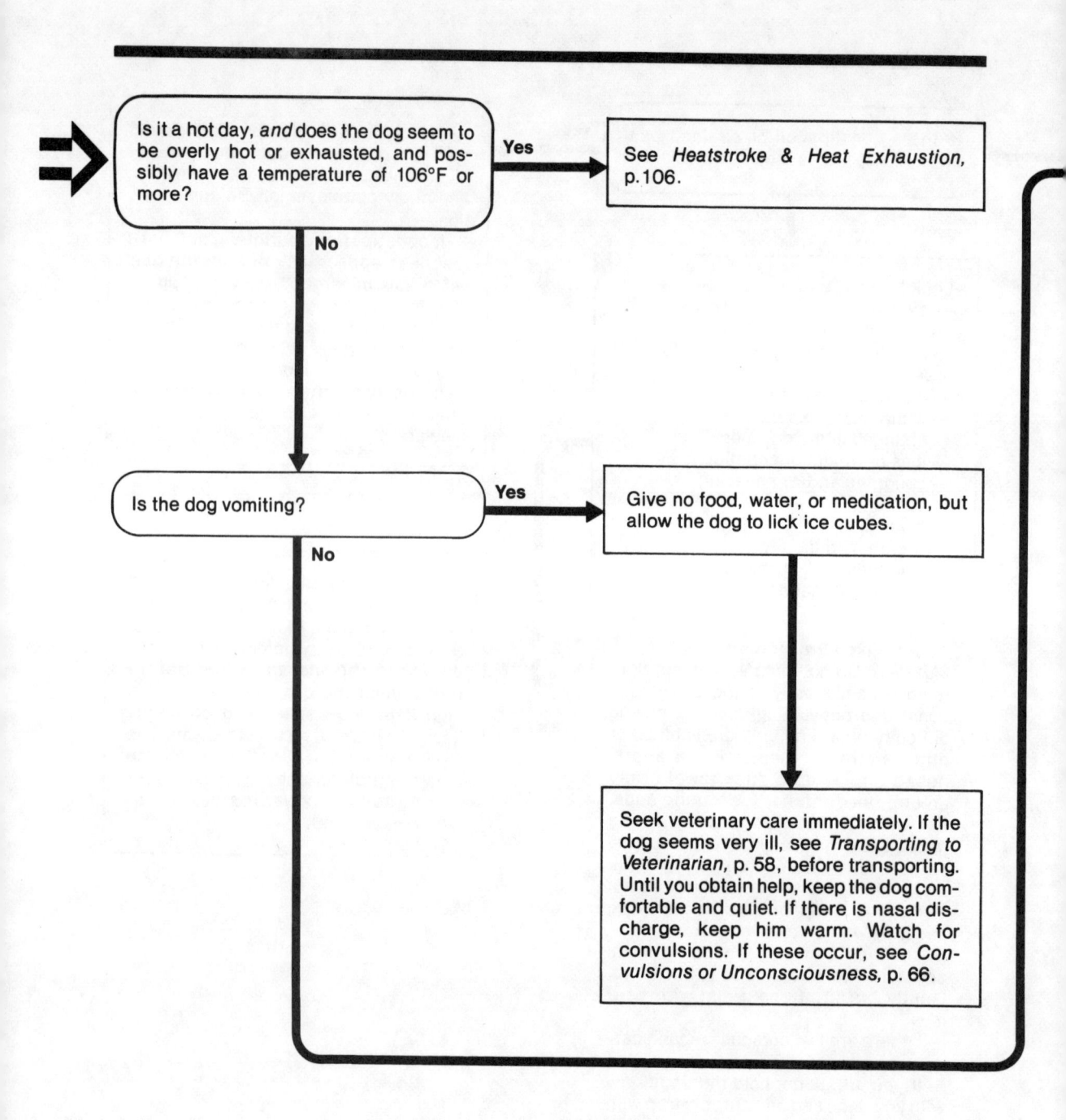

To take the dog's temperature, see p. 51.

→ Is it a hot day, *and* does the dog seem to be overly hot or exhausted, and possibly have a temperature of 106°F or more?

Yes → See *Heatstroke & Heat Exhaustion*, p. 106.

No ↓

Is the dog vomiting?

Yes → Give no food, water, or medication, but allow the dog to lick ice cubes.

↓

Seek veterinary care immediately. If the dog seems very ill, see *Transporting to Veterinarian*, p. 58, before transporting. Until you obtain help, keep the dog comfortable and quiet. If there is nasal discharge, keep him warm. Watch for convulsions. If these occur, see *Convulsions or Unconsciousness*, p. 66.

No → (proceeds to same action box)

Possible Signs & Symptoms: *temperature of 103°F or over/feels hot to the touch/shivering/loss of appetite/depression/convulsions.*

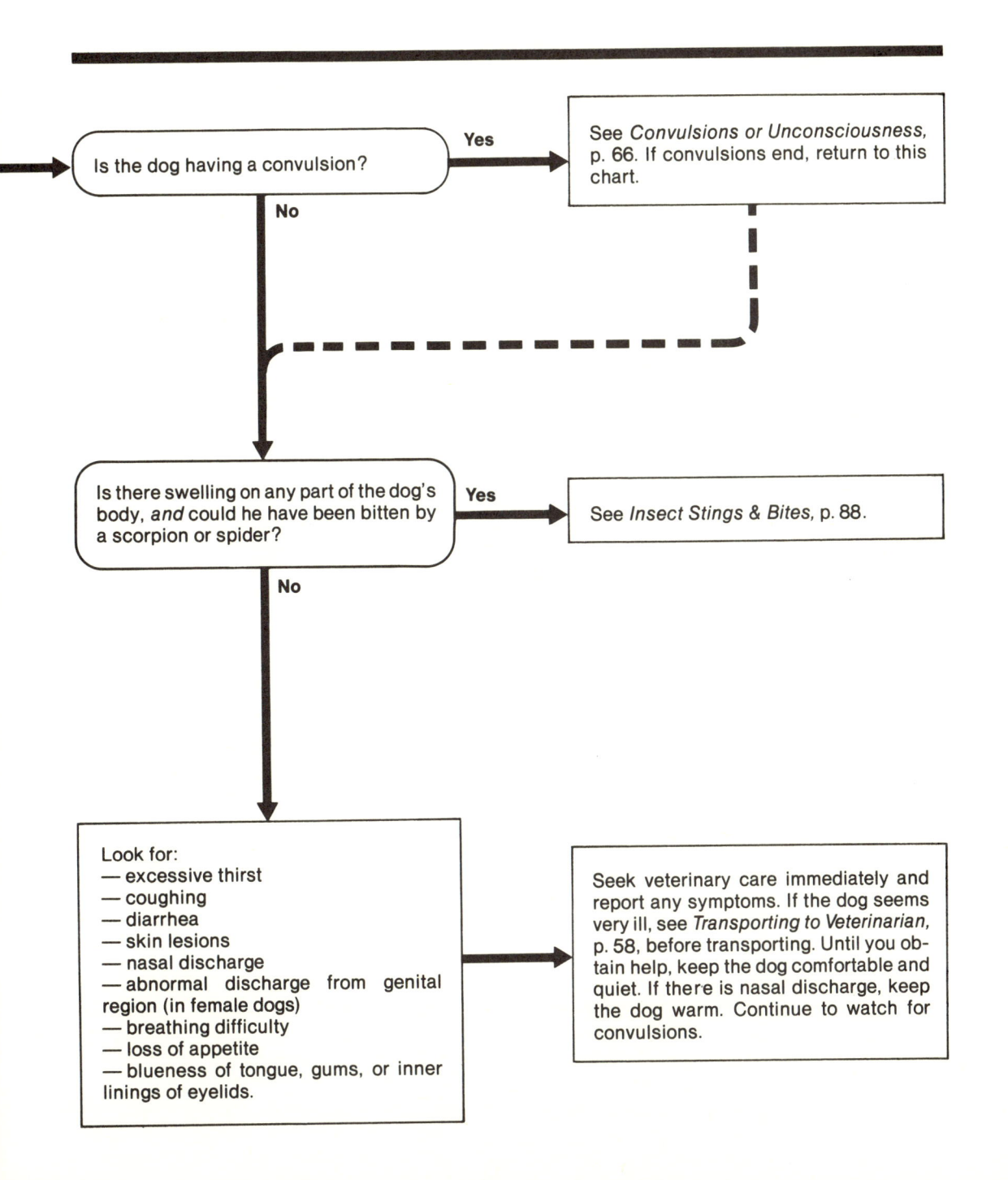

Calm the dog by speaking gently.

Is the dog having a convulsion? — **Yes** → See *Convulsions or Unconsciousness*, p. 66. If convulsions end, return to this chart.

No ↓

Is there swelling on any part of the dog's body, *and* could he have been bitten by a scorpion or spider? — **Yes** → See *Insect Stings & Bites*, p. 88.

No ↓

Look for:
— excessive thirst
— coughing
— diarrhea
— skin lesions
— nasal discharge
— abnormal discharge from genital region (in female dogs)
— breathing difficulty
— loss of appetite
— blueness of tongue, gums, or inner linings of eyelids.

→ Seek veterinary care immediately and report any symptoms. If the dog seems very ill, see *Transporting to Veterinarian*, p. 58, before transporting. Until you obtain help, keep the dog comfortable and quiet. If there is nasal discharge, keep the dog warm. Continue to watch for convulsions.

Vomiting

Try to differentiate vomiting from a gagging cough. If a cough persists, contact a veterinarian.

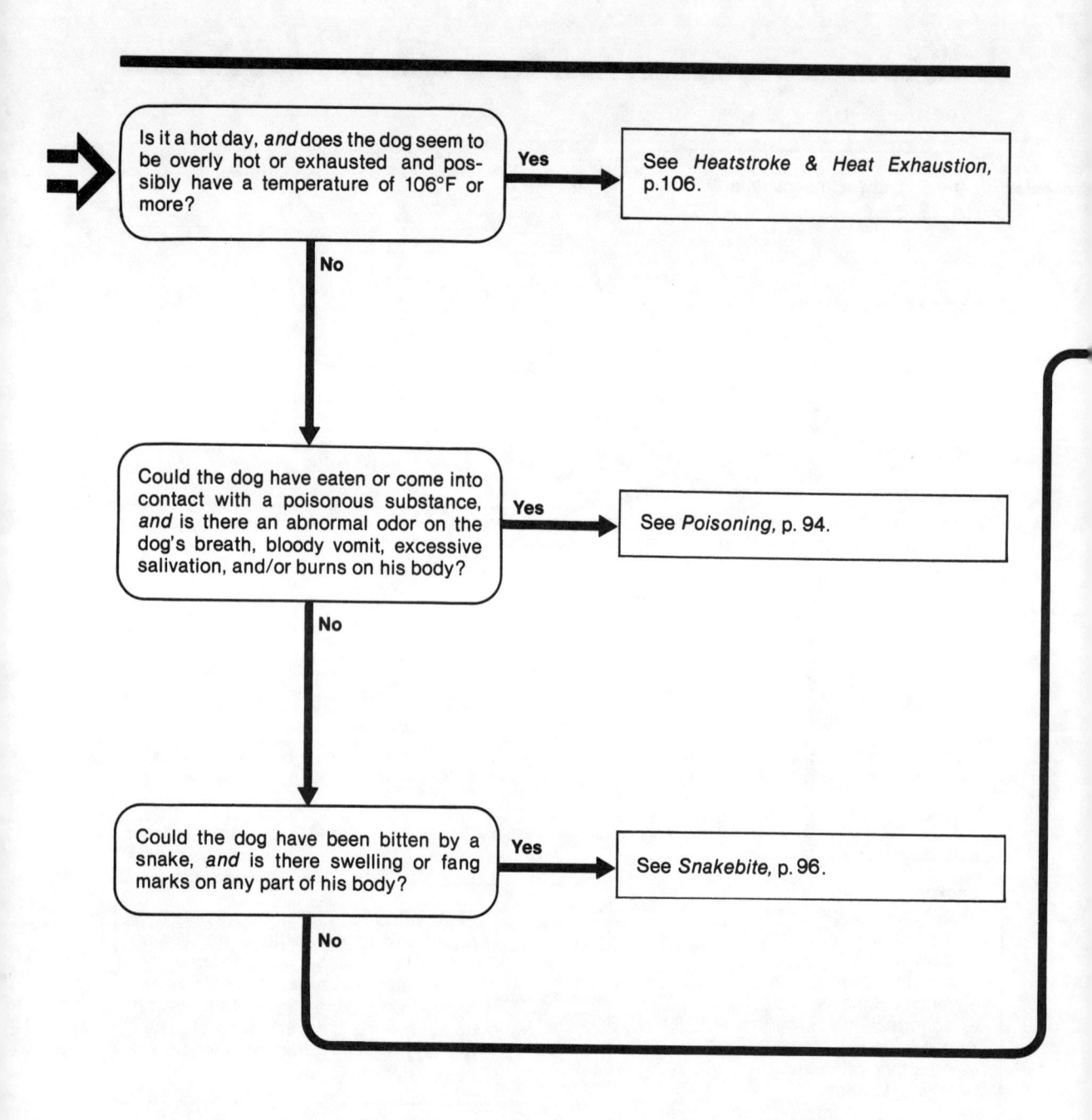

→ Is it a hot day, *and* does the dog seem to be overly hot or exhausted and possibly have a temperature of 106°F or more? — **Yes** → See *Heatstroke & Heat Exhaustion*, p.106.

↓ **No**

Could the dog have eaten or come into contact with a poisonous substance, *and* is there an abnormal odor on the dog's breath, bloody vomit, excessive salivation, and/or burns on his body? — **Yes** → See *Poisoning*, p. 94.

↓ **No**

Could the dog have been bitten by a snake, *and* is there swelling or fang marks on any part of his body? — **Yes** → See *Snakebite*, p. 96.

↓ **No**

Calm the dog by speaking gently.

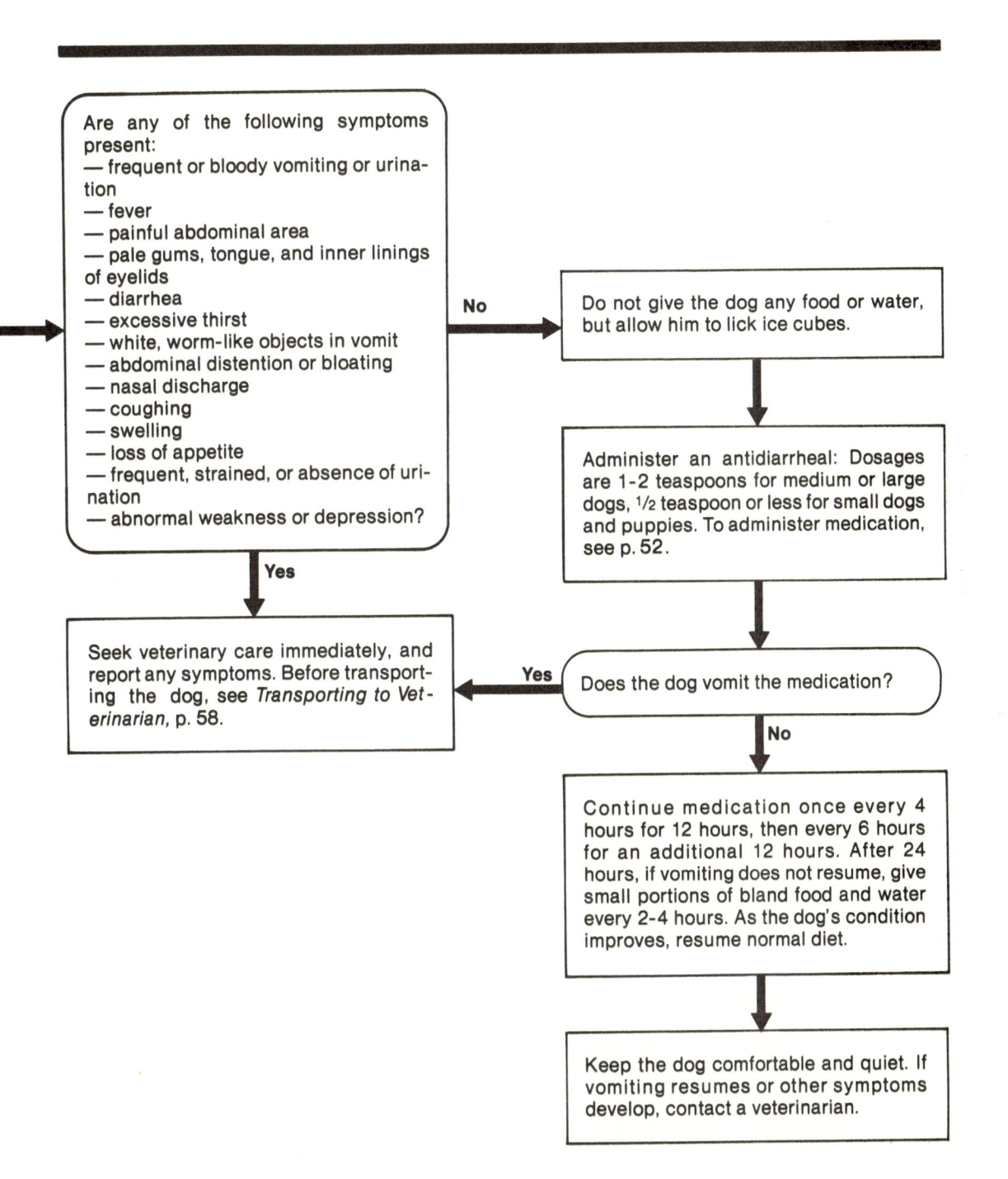

Are any of the following symptoms present:
— frequent or bloody vomiting or urination
— fever
— painful abdominal area
— pale gums, tongue, and inner linings of eyelids
— diarrhea
— excessive thirst
— white, worm-like objects in vomit
— abdominal distention or bloating
— nasal discharge
— coughing
— swelling
— loss of appetite
— frequent, strained, or absence of urination
— abnormal weakness or depression?

No → Do not give the dog any food or water, but allow him to lick ice cubes.

↓

Administer an antidiarrheal: Dosages are 1-2 teaspoons for medium or large dogs, 1/2 teaspoon or less for small dogs and puppies. To administer medication, see p. 52.

↓

Does the dog vomit the medication?

Yes ← Seek veterinary care immediately, and report any symptoms. Before transporting the dog, see *Transporting to Veterinarian*, p. 58.

Yes (from symptoms box) → Seek veterinary care immediately, and report any symptoms. Before transporting the dog, see *Transporting to Veterinarian*, p. 58.

No ↓

Continue medication once every 4 hours for 12 hours, then every 6 hours for an additional 12 hours. After 24 hours, if vomiting does not resume, give small portions of bland food and water every 2-4 hours. As the dog's condition improves, resume normal diet.

↓

Keep the dog comfortable and quiet. If vomiting resumes or other symptoms develop, contact a veterinarian.

Abdominal & Chest Injuries

Do not remove or probe for any foreign object that may have caused injury. Instead, stabilize object with clean bandages, and cover as described below.

➡ Gently restrain the dog, if necessary. (See Restraining Procedure box.) Move him if he is in an unsafe area, keeping his back and neck as straight as possible, and have him lie quietly.

Restraining Procedure:
Muzzling:* For a short-nosed dog, wrap a thick towel firmly around head and neck, securing ends. For a long-nosed dog, bring a long gauze or cloth strip under chin; make a single half-knot on top, bring back under chin, tie a single half-knot again, and bring ends behind head, tying securely with a bow. Do not knot.
Move the dog if in an unsafe area, keeping his back and neck as straight as possible.
Restraining: If the dog is not lying down, straddle his back, facing his head. Gently but firmly hold him with your legs. To have him sit, press on hind quarters; to have him lie, apply firm, gentle pressure gradually to upper back.
— If there are two persons, second person can now treat the dog.
— If you are alone, hold the dog firmly with your legs and one arm, or strap with ties, belts, etc., before treating.

Is there bleeding from the chest area, *and* does the injury appear to be a sucking wound? (Symptoms may include the sound of air being drawn through wound and/or grunting or loud breathing.)

No →

Yes ↓

— Quickly prepare dressing: Obtain a plastic bag or wrap or aluminum foil large enough to cover the entire wound. If no foil, bag, or wrap is available, cover with your hand.
— Fix any dressing tightly in place, and tape all around. Use additional dressing, if necessary, to make as airtight as possible. *Do not* apply pressure.
— Place the dog on the side on which he appears most comfortable.
— Seek veterinary care immediately. Before transporting the dog, see *Back & Neck Injuries,* p. 78. Until you obtain help, watch breathing. If it stops, see *Artificial Respiration & CPR,* p. 60.

*Do not muzzle, or if muzzled, remove immediately, if the dog is unconscious, convulsing, vomiting, having difficulty breathing, or there is blood or other matter in mouth.

Possible Signs & Symptoms: *severely painful chest or abdominal area/wounds/difficult breathing/bony protuberances under skin of chest/bleeding from ears, mouth, nose, or anus/loss of consciousness.*

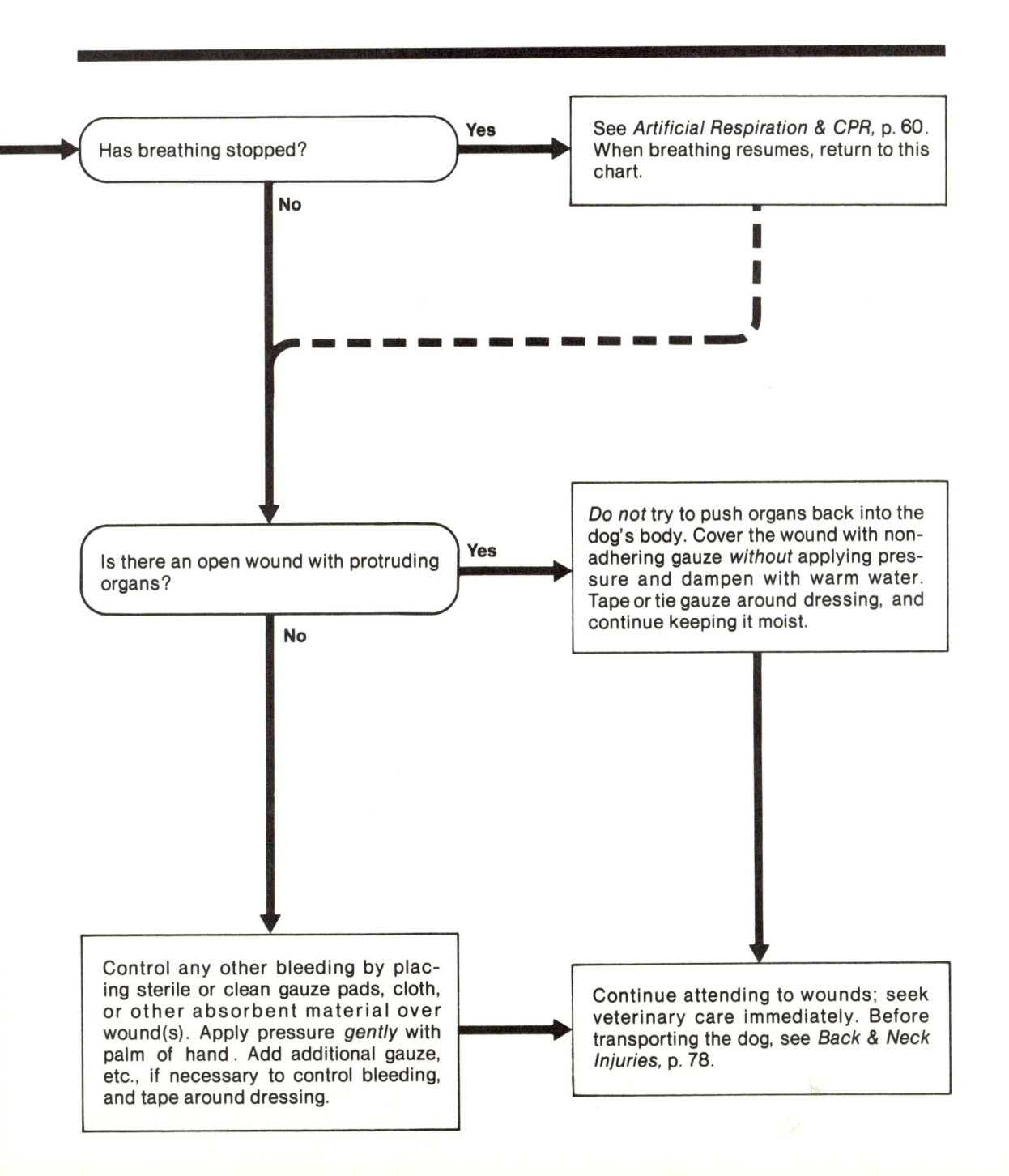

Calm the dog by speaking gently.

Has breathing stopped? — **Yes** → See *Artificial Respiration & CPR,* p. 60. When breathing resumes, return to this chart.

No ↓

Is there an open wound with protruding organs? — **Yes** → *Do not* try to push organs back into the dog's body. Cover the wound with non-adhering gauze *without* applying pressure and dampen with warm water. Tape or tie gauze around dressing, and continue keeping it moist.

No ↓

Control any other bleeding by placing sterile or clean gauze pads, cloth, or other absorbent material over wound(s). Apply pressure *gently* with palm of hand. Add additional gauze, etc., if necessary to control bleeding, and tape around dressing.

→ Continue attending to wounds; seek veterinary care immediately. Before transporting the dog, see *Back & Neck Injuries,* p. 78.

Allergic Reaction

If you suspect food poisoning, see *Poisoning*, p. 94. Symptoms may include vomiting, diarrhea, and/or painful abdominal area.

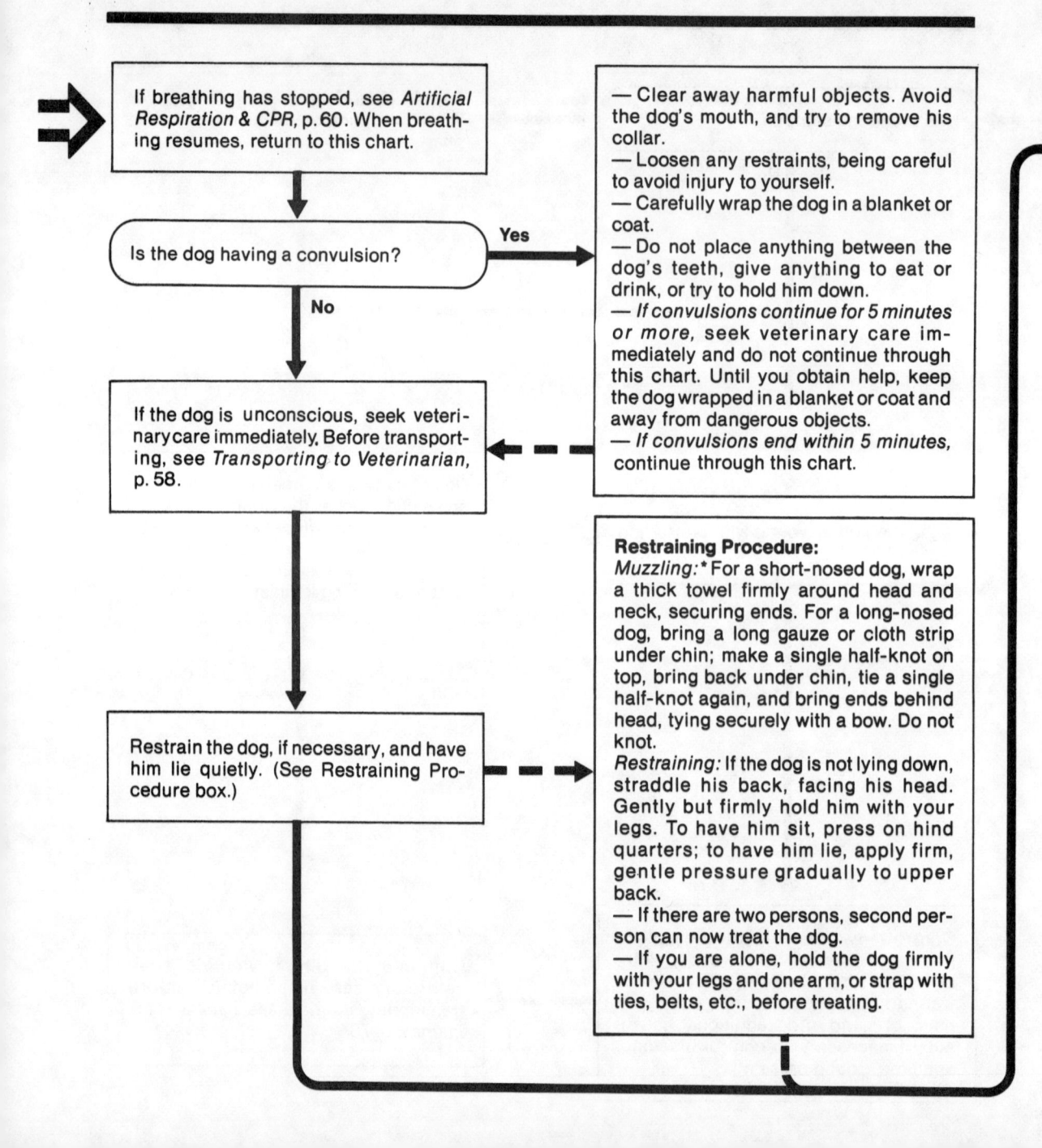

→ If breathing has stopped, see *Artificial Respiration & CPR*, p. 60. When breathing resumes, return to this chart.

↓

Is the dog having a convulsion? — **Yes** →
- Clear away harmful objects. Avoid the dog's mouth, and try to remove his collar.
- Loosen any restraints, being careful to avoid injury to yourself.
- Carefully wrap the dog in a blanket or coat.
- Do not place anything between the dog's teeth, give anything to eat or drink, or try to hold him down.
- *If convulsions continue for 5 minutes or more,* seek veterinary care immediately and do not continue through this chart. Until you obtain help, keep the dog wrapped in a blanket or coat and away from dangerous objects.
- *If convulsions end within 5 minutes,* continue through this chart.

No ↓

If the dog is unconscious, seek veterinary care immediately. Before transporting, see *Transporting to Veterinarian*, p. 58. ◀---

↓

Restrain the dog, if necessary, and have him lie quietly. (See Restraining Procedure box.) ---▶

Restraining Procedure:
Muzzling: * For a short-nosed dog, wrap a thick towel firmly around head and neck, securing ends. For a long-nosed dog, bring a long gauze or cloth strip under chin; make a single half-knot on top, bring back under chin, tie a single half-knot again, and bring ends behind head, tying securely with a bow. Do not knot.
Restraining: If the dog is not lying down, straddle his back, facing his head. Gently but firmly hold him with your legs. To have him sit, press on hind quarters; to have him lie, apply firm, gentle pressure gradually to upper back.
- If there are two persons, second person can now treat the dog.
- If you are alone, hold the dog firmly with your legs and one arm, or strap with ties, belts, etc., before treating.

Possible Signs & Symptoms: *swelling/itching/ hives/ panting/ difficult breathing/ convulsions/ loss of consciousness.*

Calm the dog by speaking gently.

If the dog is more than 8 weeks old and not pregnant, give an antihistamine — 1-2 teaspoons or tablets for medium or large dogs, 1/2 teaspoon or tablet or less for small dogs. To administer medication, see p. 52.

Was the reaction caused by a drug injection or insect sting?

Yes →

— Place the dog so that the sting or bite site is below heart level or, if not possible, at the same level.
— If wound is on a leg, tie a 1" wide cloth strip or handkerchief snugly 2"-4" above wound (not on a joint), leaving it loose enough to slip one finger underneath. (See illustration below.)
— Cut hair around the wound and gently wash with mild soap and water; rinse well.
— If a stinger or venom sac is present, carefully scrape it off using a clean fingernail, tweezers, knife, or razor blade. *Do not* cut skin or squeeze stinger or sac.
— Apply ice pack to wound site. Try not to cause cold injury.

No ↓

Seek veterinary care immediately. Before transporting the dog, see *Transporting to Veterinarian,* p. 58. Loosen any constricting band briefly every 3-5 minutes. Until you obtain help, if the dog is conscious with *no* vomiting or convulsions, give small amounts of non-alcoholic liquids to drink. Continue to check for convulsions.

*Do not muzzle, or if muzzled, remove immediately, if the dog is unconscious, convulsing, vomiting, having difficulty breathing, or there is blood or other matter in mouth.

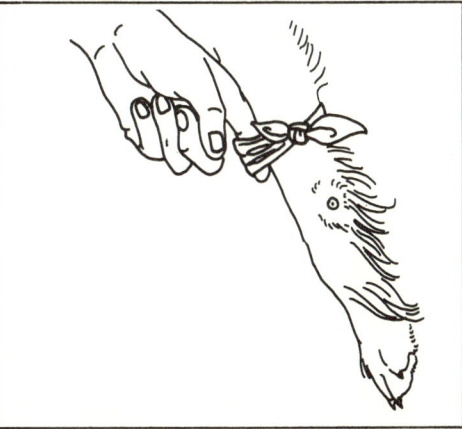

Back & Neck Injuries

Attend to any other injuries before using this chart: *Head & Facial Injuries*, p. 86; *Abdominal & Chest Injuries*, p. 74; *Leg Fractures, Sprains & Dislocations*, p. 90; *Puncture & Deep Wounds*, p.102; *Eye Injuries*, p. 84.

With any severe back injury, assume fracture of both neck and back.

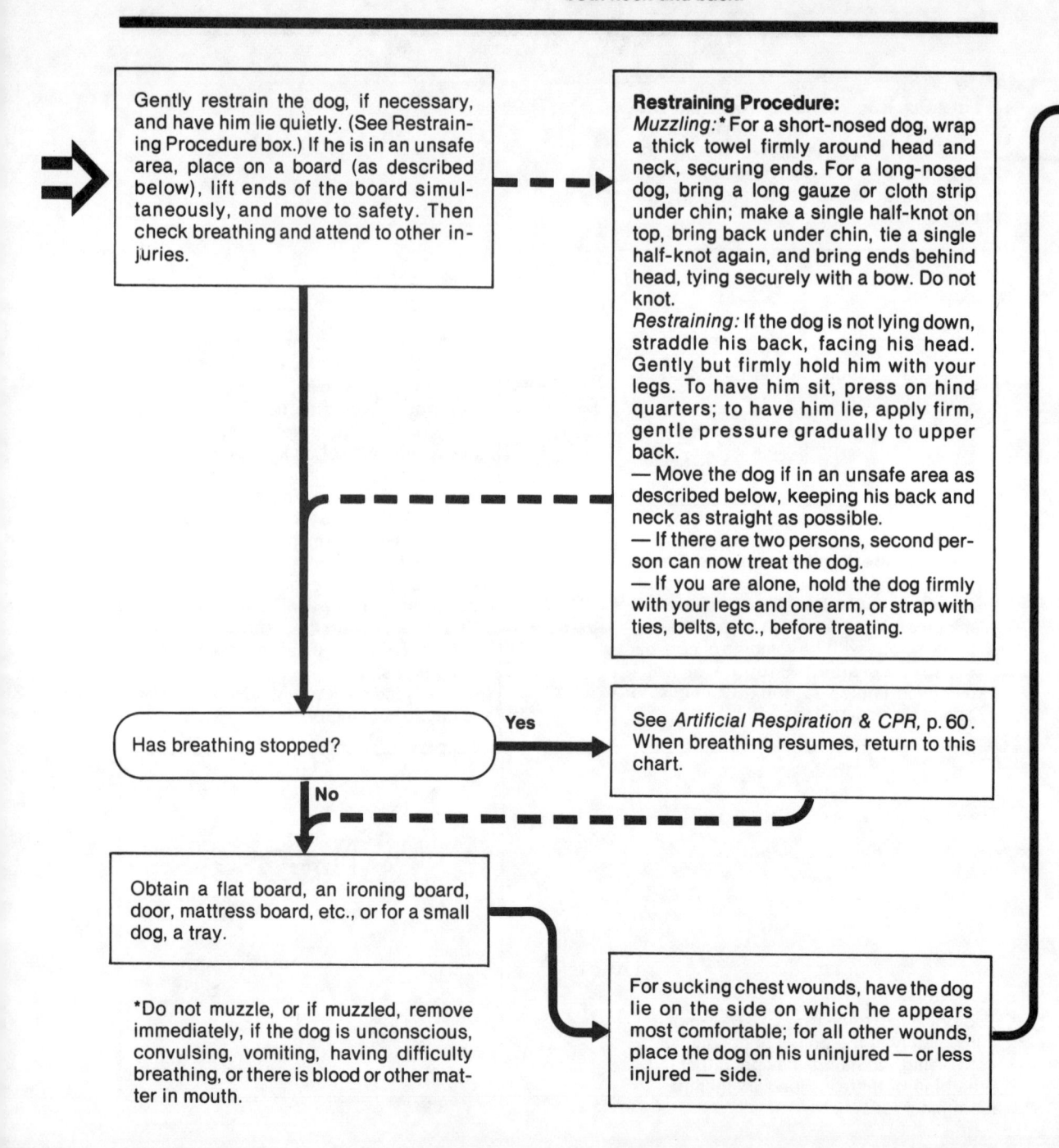

→ Gently restrain the dog, if necessary, and have him lie quietly. (See Restraining Procedure box.) If he is in an unsafe area, place on a board (as described below), lift ends of the board simultaneously, and move to safety. Then check breathing and attend to other injuries.

Restraining Procedure:
*Muzzling:** For a short-nosed dog, wrap a thick towel firmly around head and neck, securing ends. For a long-nosed dog, bring a long gauze or cloth strip under chin; make a single half-knot on top, bring back under chin, tie a single half-knot again, and bring ends behind head, tying securely with a bow. Do not knot.
Restraining: If the dog is not lying down, straddle his back, facing his head. Gently but firmly hold him with your legs. To have him sit, press on hind quarters; to have him lie, apply firm, gentle pressure gradually to upper back.
— Move the dog if in an unsafe area as described below, keeping his back and neck as straight as possible.
— If there are two persons, second person can now treat the dog.
— If you are alone, hold the dog firmly with your legs and one arm, or strap with ties, belts, etc., before treating.

Has breathing stopped? — **Yes** → See *Artificial Respiration & CPR*, p. 60. When breathing resumes, return to this chart.

No ↓

Obtain a flat board, an ironing board, door, mattress board, etc., or for a small dog, a tray.

For sucking chest wounds, have the dog lie on the side on which he appears most comfortable; for all other wounds, place the dog on his uninjured — or less injured — side.

*Do not muzzle, or if muzzled, remove immediately, if the dog is unconscious, convulsing, vomiting, having difficulty breathing, or there is blood or other matter in mouth.

Possible Signs & Symptoms: *pain at site of injury/deformity or swelling of injured area/paralysis of or lack of sensation in one or more legs/loss of strength/rigidity of front legs/difficult breathing/loss of bowel and bladder control/loss of consciousness.*

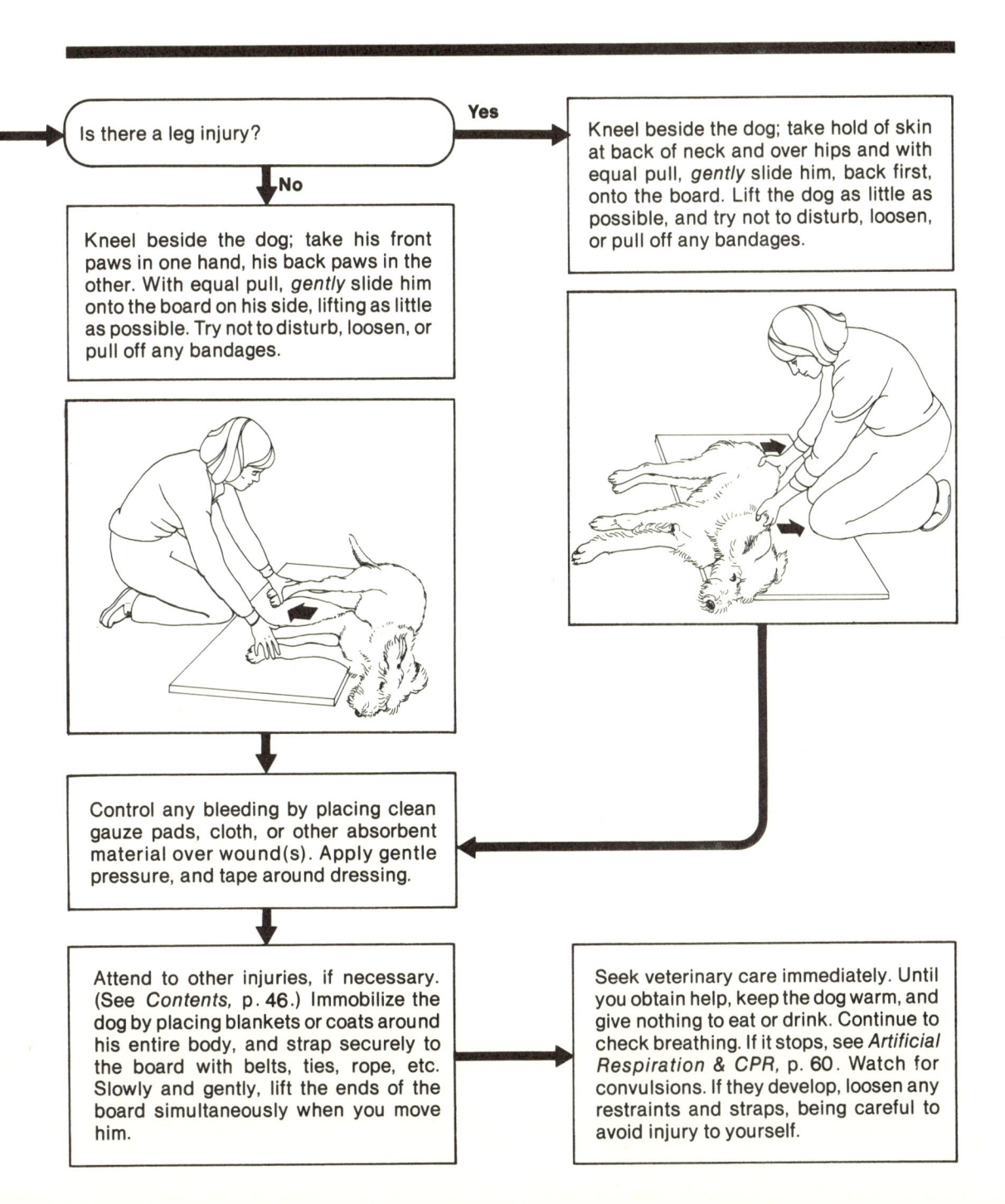

Calm the dog by speaking gently.

Is there a leg injury? → **Yes** → Kneel beside the dog; take hold of skin at back of neck and over hips and with equal pull, *gently* slide him, back first, onto the board. Lift the dog as little as possible, and try not to disturb, loosen, or pull off any bandages.

↓ No

Kneel beside the dog; take his front paws in one hand, his back paws in the other. With equal pull, *gently* slide him onto the board on his side, lifting as little as possible. Try not to disturb, loosen, or pull off any bandages.

Control any bleeding by placing clean gauze pads, cloth, or other absorbent material over wound(s). Apply gentle pressure, and tape around dressing.

Attend to other injuries, if necessary. (See *Contents,* p. 46.) Immobilize the dog by placing blankets or coats around his entire body, and strap securely to the board with belts, ties, rope, etc. Slowly and gently, lift the ends of the board simultaneously when you move him.

Seek veterinary care immediately. Until you obtain help, keep the dog warm, and give nothing to eat or drink. Continue to check breathing. If it stops, see *Artificial Respiration & CPR,* p. 60. Watch for convulsions. If they develop, loosen any restraints and straps, being careful to avoid injury to yourself.

Burns
(Including Electric Shock & Chemical Burns)

Do not attempt to clean off any dead skin from burn, break blisters, or give medication.

→ If the dog is unconscious, check breathing. If it has stopped, see *Artificial Respiration & CPR*, p. 60. When breathing resumes, return to this chart.

→ Restrain the dog, if necessary. (See Restraining Procedure box.) Gently move him if he is in an unsafe area. If anything is sticking to burn(s), do not attempt to remove it.

Restraining Procedure:
Muzzling: For a short-nosed dog, wrap a thick towel firmly around head and neck, securing ends. For a long-nosed dog, bring a long gauze or cloth strip under chin; make a single half-knot on top, bring back under chin, tie a single half-knot again, and bring ends behind head, tying securely into a bow. Do not knot.
Move the dog if in an unsafe area.
Restraining: If the dog is not lying down, straddle his back, facing his head. Gently but firmly hold him with your legs. To have him sit, press on hind quarters; to have him lie, apply firm, gentle pressure gradually to upper back.
— If there are two persons, second person can now treat the dog.
— If you are alone, hold the dog firmly with your legs and one arm, or strap with ties, belts, etc., before treating.

First Degree

Apply cold, wet compresses to the burned area, or immerse the burn in fresh, cold water — not ice or salt water.

The skin should heal in a short time. If it does not, contact a veterinarian.

Continue cold water applications until pain appears to subside (usually about 5-10 minutes). Leave uncovered, if possible, or lightly cover entirely with dry, non-adhering gauze, and tape around dressing.

→ Are burns due to electric shock? **No** / **Yes**

Possible Signs & Symptoms:
First Degree: *singed hair/redness of skin/pain, with mild swelling.*
Second Degree: *burned-off hair/deep redness of skin with severe swelling/glossy appearance from leaking fluid/blisters or skin loss.*
Third Degree: *complete loss of hair/painless/white or blackish skin. This is a very serious type of burn.*

In cases of electric shock, if the dog is still touching the electric source, do not touch either the dog or the source. First, **turn off the master electrical switch**, or **pull the appliance plug**. If caused by a fallen electric wire, do not try to move the wire away. Instead, obtain emergency assistance (i.e., police, fire department, etc.).

Calm the dog by speaking gently.

Has the dog been burned by a chemical? — **Yes** → Put on rubber gloves, then flush the burned area (including mouth and eyes, if necessary) with cool water for at least 5 minutes. Be sure to wash chemical away completely. Cover burns lightly with clean, non-adhering gauze. Tape or tie gauze bandages gently around dressing. Seek veterinary care immediately. Before transporting the dog, see *Transporting to Veterinarian*, p. 58. Until you obtain help, if vomiting or diarrhea is present, see *Poisoning*, p. 94.

No ↓

Based on the Possible Signs & Symptoms listed above, determine whether the burn is first, second, or third degree. If you're in doubt or if the burn is extensive, choose the more serious classification.

Second Degree

Immerse the burn in fresh, cold water — not ice or salt water — or apply cold, wet compresses. Continue for 10-15 minutes.

↓

Gently dry with sterile gauze or clean cloth and lightly cover the burn entirely with dry, non-adhering gauze.

Third Degree

Lightly cover the burn entirely with non-adhering gauze. (Do not use material that can leave lint in burn.) *Do not* use wet compresses and *do not* immerse the burn in water.

↓

Continue to check breathing, and seek veterinary care immediately. Before transporting the dog, see *Transporting to Veterinarian*, p. 58.

*Do not muzzle, or if muzzled, remove immediately, if the dog is unconscious, convulsing, vomiting, having difficulty breathing, or there is blood or other matter in mouth.

Minor Cuts & Scratches
(Including Minor Animal Bites)

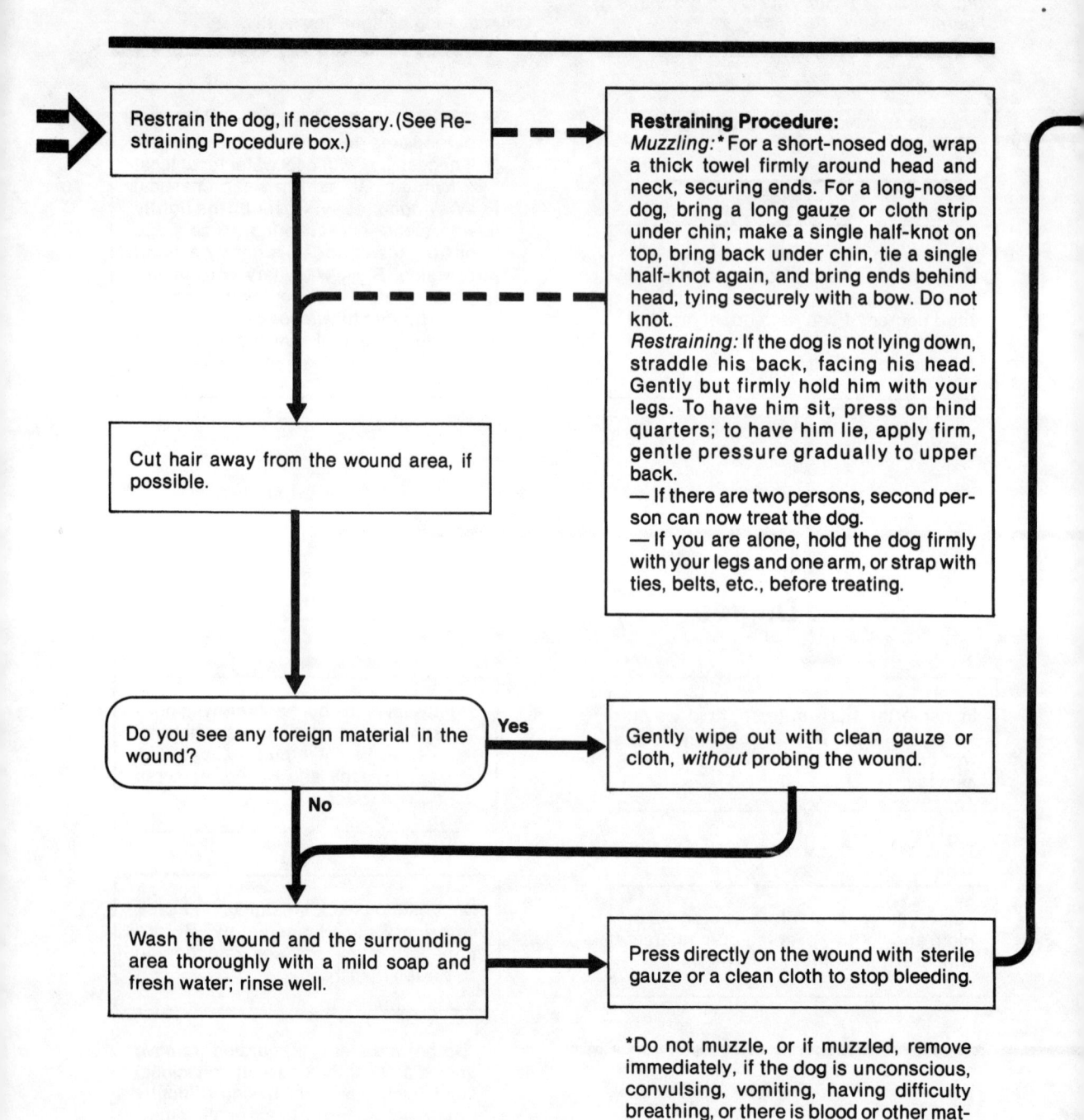

→ Restrain the dog, if necessary. (See Restraining Procedure box.)

Restraining Procedure:
Muzzling:* For a short-nosed dog, wrap a thick towel firmly around head and neck, securing ends. For a long-nosed dog, bring a long gauze or cloth strip under chin; make a single half-knot on top, bring back under chin, tie a single half-knot again, and bring ends behind head, tying securely with a bow. Do not knot.
Restraining: If the dog is not lying down, straddle his back, facing his head. Gently but firmly hold him with your legs. To have him sit, press on hind quarters; to have him lie, apply firm, gentle pressure gradually to upper back.
— If there are two persons, second person can now treat the dog.
— If you are alone, hold the dog firmly with your legs and one arm, or strap with ties, belts, etc., before treating.

Cut hair away from the wound area, if possible.

Do you see any foreign material in the wound?

Yes → Gently wipe out with clean gauze or cloth, *without* probing the wound.

No ↓

Wash the wound and the surrounding area thoroughly with a mild soap and fresh water; rinse well.

Press directly on the wound with sterile gauze or a clean cloth to stop bleeding.

*Do not muzzle, or if muzzled, remove immediately, if the dog is unconscious, convulsing, vomiting, having difficulty breathing, or there is blood or other matter in mouth.

Calm the dog by speaking gently.

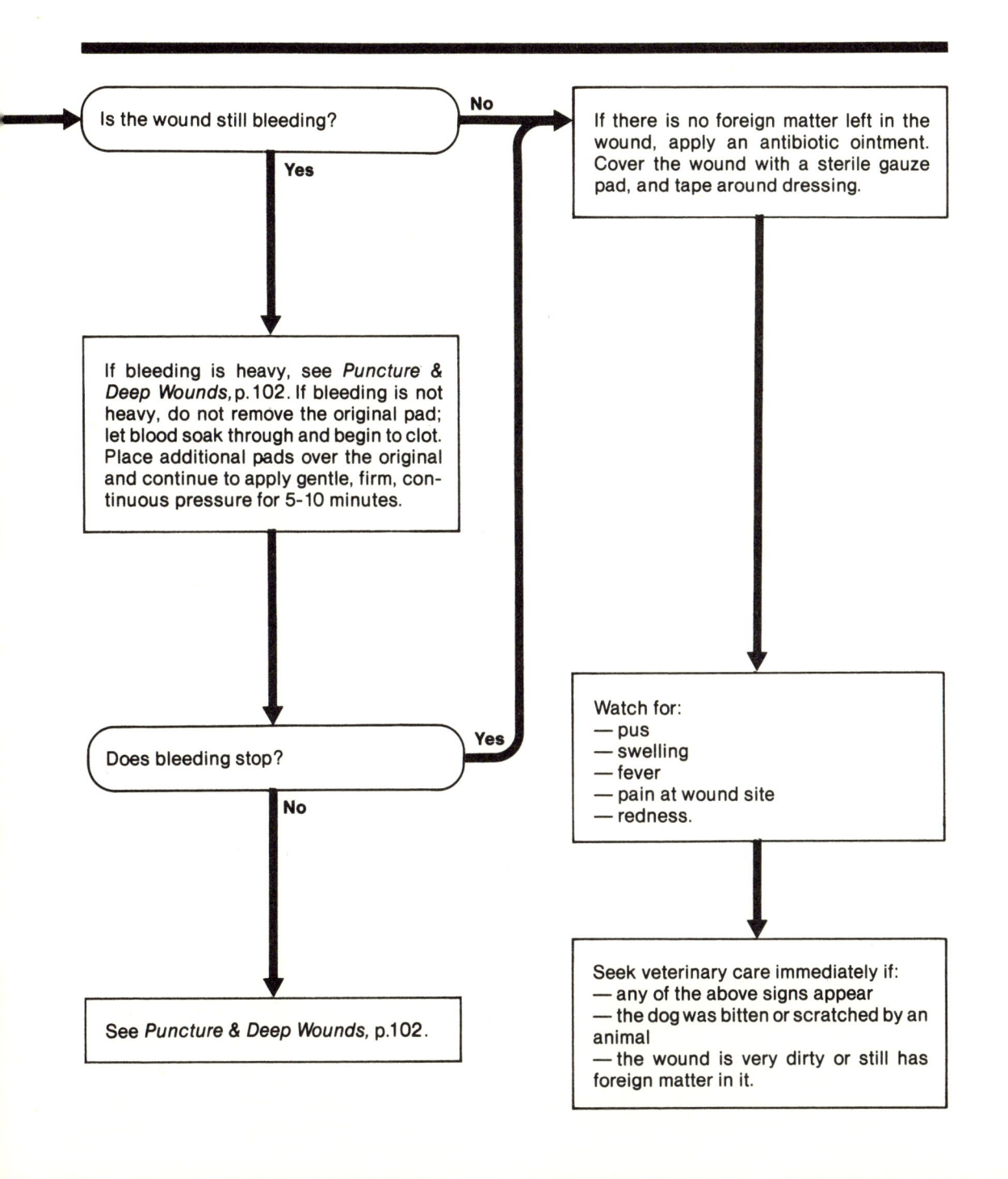

→ Is the wound still bleeding? —No→ If there is no foreign matter left in the wound, apply an antibiotic ointment. Cover the wound with a sterile gauze pad, and tape around dressing.

↓ Yes

If bleeding is heavy, see *Puncture & Deep Wounds*, p.102. If bleeding is not heavy, do not remove the original pad; let blood soak through and begin to clot. Place additional pads over the original and continue to apply gentle, firm, continuous pressure for 5-10 minutes.

↓

Does bleeding stop? —Yes→

↓ No

See *Puncture & Deep Wounds*, p.102.

Watch for:
— pus
— swelling
— fever
— pain at wound site
— redness.

↓

Seek veterinary care immediately if:
— any of the above signs appear
— the dog was bitten or scratched by an animal
— the wound is very dirty or still has foreign matter in it.

Eye Injuries
(Including Foreign Object & Chemical Burns)

Dogs have what is called a "third eyelid," located at the inner corner of the eye, which can expand over the eye after injury. If this occurs, do not treat or touch the eye, but seek veterinary care immediately.

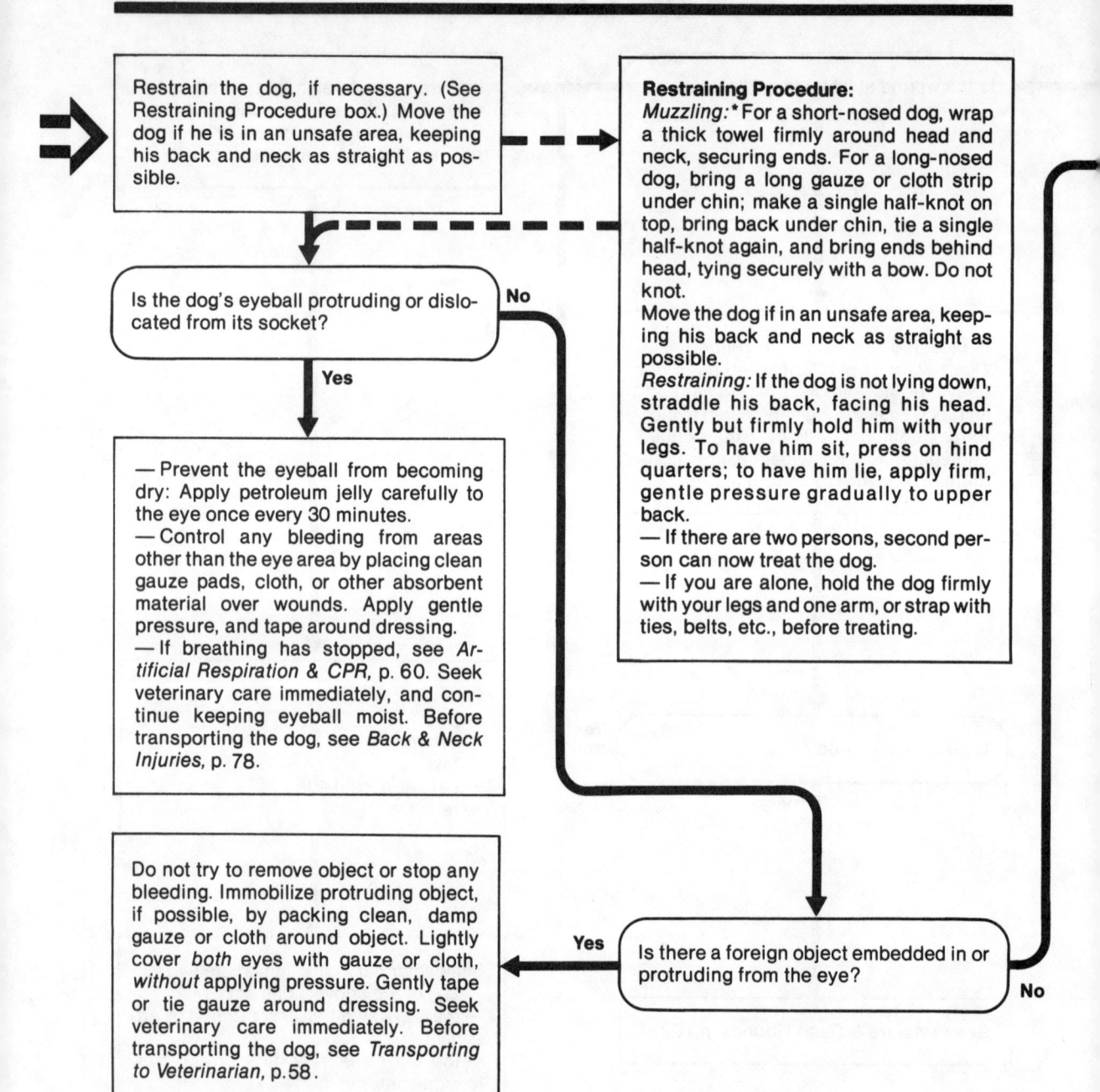

Restrain the dog, if necessary. (See Restraining Procedure box.) Move the dog if he is in an unsafe area, keeping his back and neck as straight as possible.

Restraining Procedure:
*Muzzling:** For a short-nosed dog, wrap a thick towel firmly around head and neck, securing ends. For a long-nosed dog, bring a long gauze or cloth strip under chin; make a single half-knot on top, bring back under chin, tie a single half-knot again, and bring ends behind head, tying securely with a bow. Do not knot.

Move the dog if in an unsafe area, keeping his back and neck as straight as possible.

Restraining: If the dog is not lying down, straddle his back, facing his head. Gently but firmly hold him with your legs. To have him sit, press on hind quarters; to have him lie, apply firm, gentle pressure gradually to upper back.

— If there are two persons, second person can now treat the dog.
— If you are alone, hold the dog firmly with your legs and one arm, or strap with ties, belts, etc., before treating.

Is the dog's eyeball protruding or dislocated from its socket?

Yes:
— Prevent the eyeball from becoming dry: Apply petroleum jelly carefully to the eye once every 30 minutes.
— Control any bleeding from areas other than the eye area by placing clean gauze pads, cloth, or other absorbent material over wounds. Apply gentle pressure, and tape around dressing.
— If breathing has stopped, see *Artificial Respiration & CPR,* p. 60. Seek veterinary care immediately, and continue keeping eyeball moist. Before transporting the dog, see *Back & Neck Injuries,* p. 78.

Is there a foreign object embedded in or protruding from the eye?

Yes:
Do not try to remove object or stop any bleeding. Immobilize protruding object, if possible, by packing clean, damp gauze or cloth around object. Lightly cover *both* eyes with gauze or cloth, *without* applying pressure. Gently tape or tie gauze around dressing. Seek veterinary care immediately. Before transporting the dog, see *Transporting to Veterinarian,* p. 58.

---

*Do not muzzle, or if muzzled, remove immediately, if the dog is unconscious, convulsing, vomiting, having difficulty breathing, or there is blood or other matter in mouth.

Possible Signs & Symptoms: *obvious foreign object in eye/protruding or dislocated eyeball/ oozing of eye contents/bleeding/tightly closed eyes / swelling / painful eye area / redness or other color changes/squinting/tearing/pawing at face or eye. Similar symptoms may indicate an eye disease or infection.*

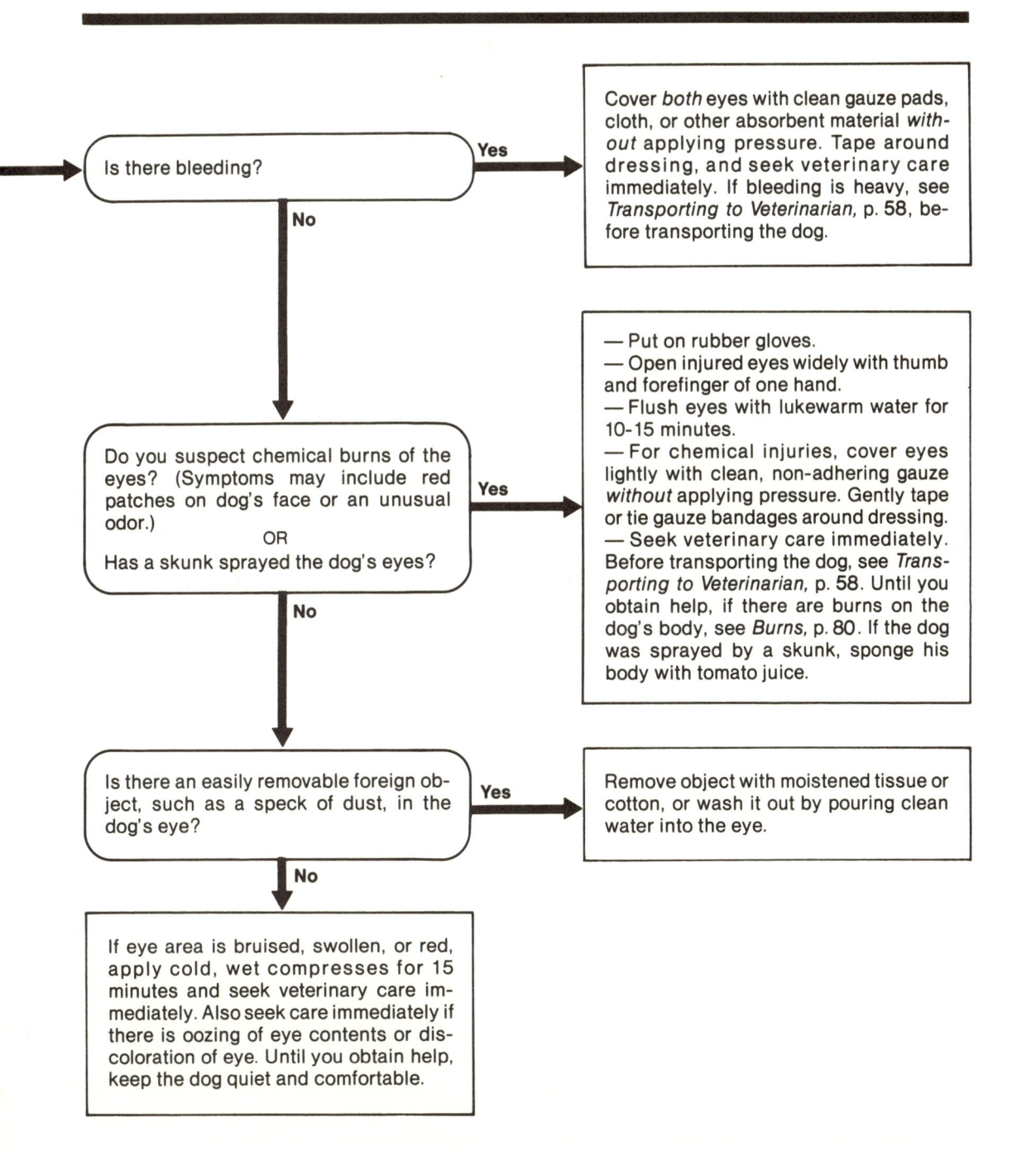

Calm the dog by speaking gently.

Is there bleeding? → **Yes** → Cover *both* eyes with clean gauze pads, cloth, or other absorbent material *without* applying pressure. Tape around dressing, and seek veterinary care immediately. If bleeding is heavy, see *Transporting to Veterinarian,* p. 58, before transporting the dog.

↓ No

Do you suspect chemical burns of the eyes? (Symptoms may include red patches on dog's face or an unusual odor.)
OR
Has a skunk sprayed the dog's eyes? → **Yes** →
— Put on rubber gloves.
— Open injured eyes widely with thumb and forefinger of one hand.
— Flush eyes with lukewarm water for 10-15 minutes.
— For chemical injuries, cover eyes lightly with clean, non-adhering gauze *without* applying pressure. Gently tape or tie gauze bandages around dressing.
— Seek veterinary care immediately. Before transporting the dog, see *Transporting to Veterinarian,* p. 58. Until you obtain help, if there are burns on the dog's body, see *Burns,* p. 80. If the dog was sprayed by a skunk, sponge his body with tomato juice.

↓ No

Is there an easily removable foreign object, such as a speck of dust, in the dog's eye? → **Yes** → Remove object with moistened tissue or cotton, or wash it out by pouring clean water into the eye.

↓ No

If eye area is bruised, swollen, or red, apply cold, wet compresses for 15 minutes and seek veterinary care immediately. Also seek care immediately if there is oozing of eye contents or discoloration of eye. Until you obtain help, keep the dog quiet and comfortable.

Head & Facial Injuries

If there is a simple nosebleed or a tooth or mouth injury, and you do *not* suspect severe head injury, see appropriate chart: *Nose Problems*, p. 92, or *Tooth & Mouth Injuries*, p. 100.

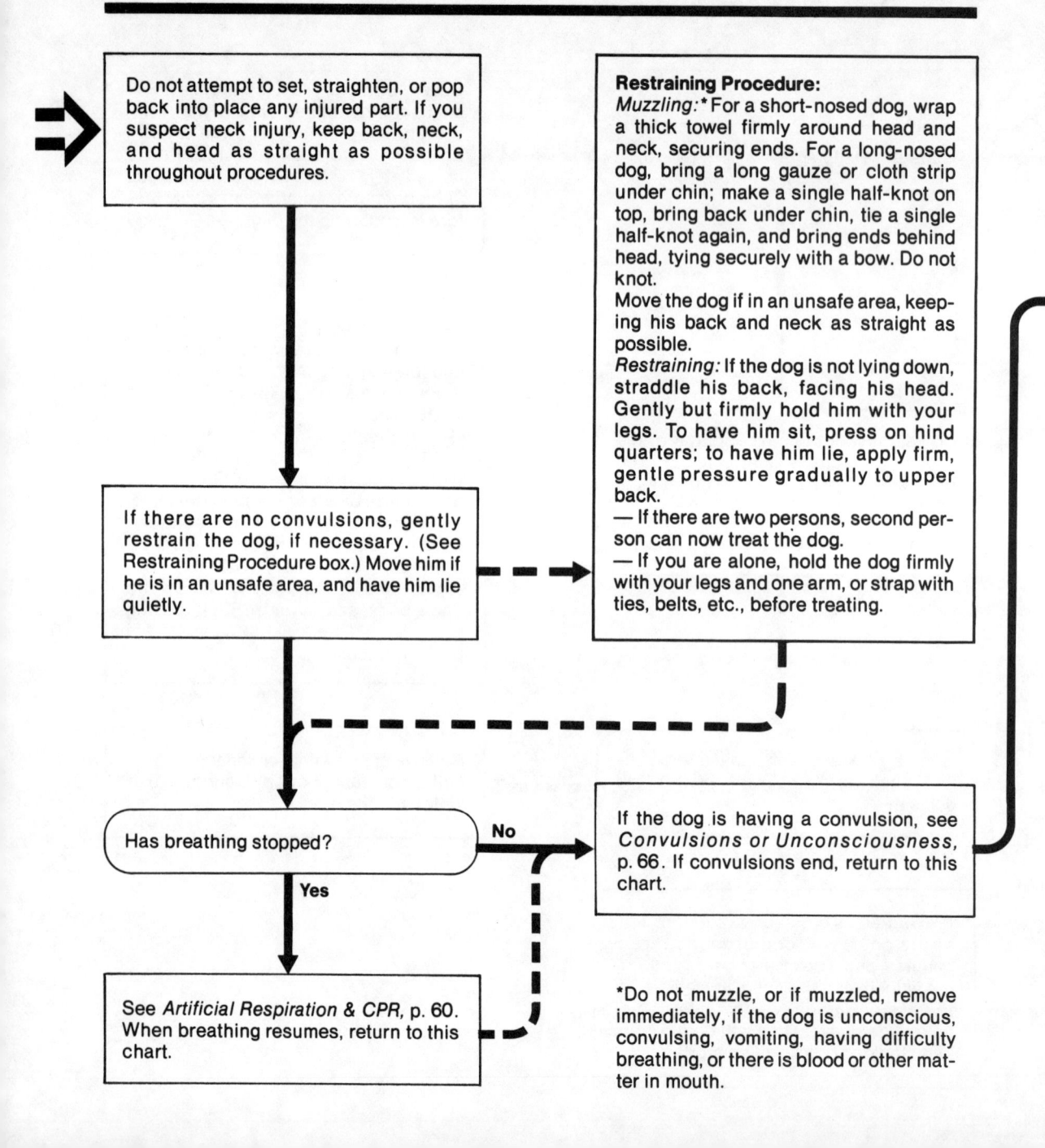

→ Do not attempt to set, straighten, or pop back into place any injured part. If you suspect neck injury, keep back, neck, and head as straight as possible throughout procedures.

↓

If there are no convulsions, gently restrain the dog, if necessary. (See Restraining Procedure box.) Move him if he is in an unsafe area, and have him lie quietly.

↓

Has breathing stopped?

Yes ↓

See *Artificial Respiration & CPR*, p. 60. When breathing resumes, return to this chart.

No →

If the dog is having a convulsion, see *Convulsions or Unconsciousness*, p. 66. If convulsions end, return to this chart.

Restraining Procedure:

Muzzling:* For a short-nosed dog, wrap a thick towel firmly around head and neck, securing ends. For a long-nosed dog, bring a long gauze or cloth strip under chin; make a single half-knot on top, bring back under chin, tie a single half-knot again, and bring ends behind head, tying securely with a bow. Do not knot.

Move the dog if in an unsafe area, keeping his back and neck as straight as possible.

Restraining: If the dog is not lying down, straddle his back, facing his head. Gently but firmly hold him with your legs. To have him sit, press on hind quarters; to have him lie, apply firm, gentle pressure gradually to upper back.

— If there are two persons, second person can now treat the dog.
— If you are alone, hold the dog firmly with your legs and one arm, or strap with ties, belts, etc., before treating.

---

*Do not muzzle, or if muzzled, remove immediately, if the dog is unconscious, convulsing, vomiting, having difficulty breathing, or there is blood or other matter in mouth.

Possible Signs & Symptoms: *bleeding or draining of clear fluid from ears, nose, or mouth/ vomiting/loss of bowel and bladder control/ pupils of unequal size/swelling/pale gums/ deformity/paralysis/convulsions/loss of consciousness.*

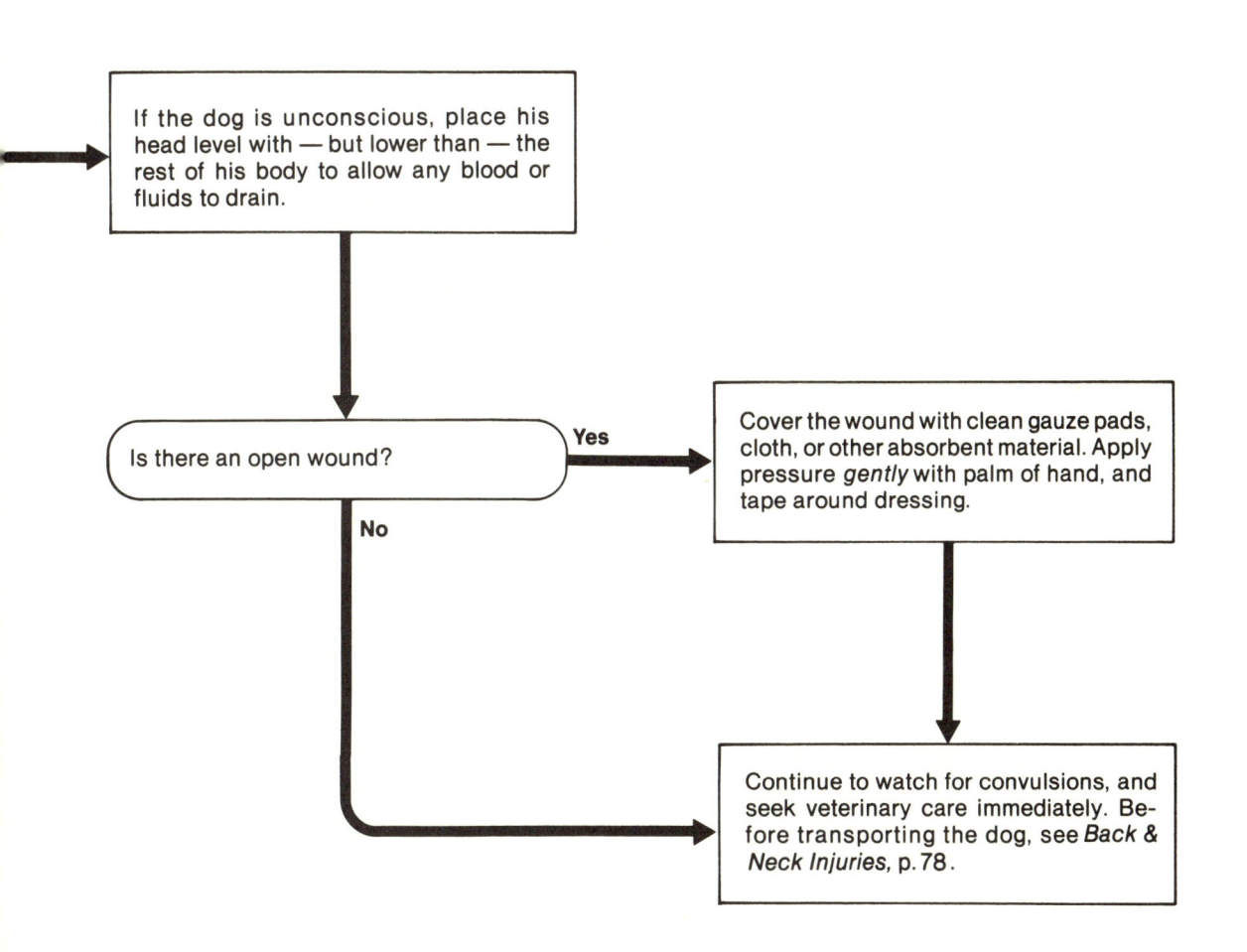

Calm the dog by speaking gently.

If the dog is unconscious, place his head level with — but lower than — the rest of his body to allow any blood or fluids to drain.

Is there an open wound?

Yes → Cover the wound with clean gauze pads, cloth, or other absorbent material. Apply pressure *gently* with palm of hand, and tape around dressing.

No ↓

Continue to watch for convulsions, and seek veterinary care immediately. Before transporting the dog, see *Back & Neck Injuries*, p. 78.

Insect Stings & Bites
(Including Spiders, Scorpions & Ticks)

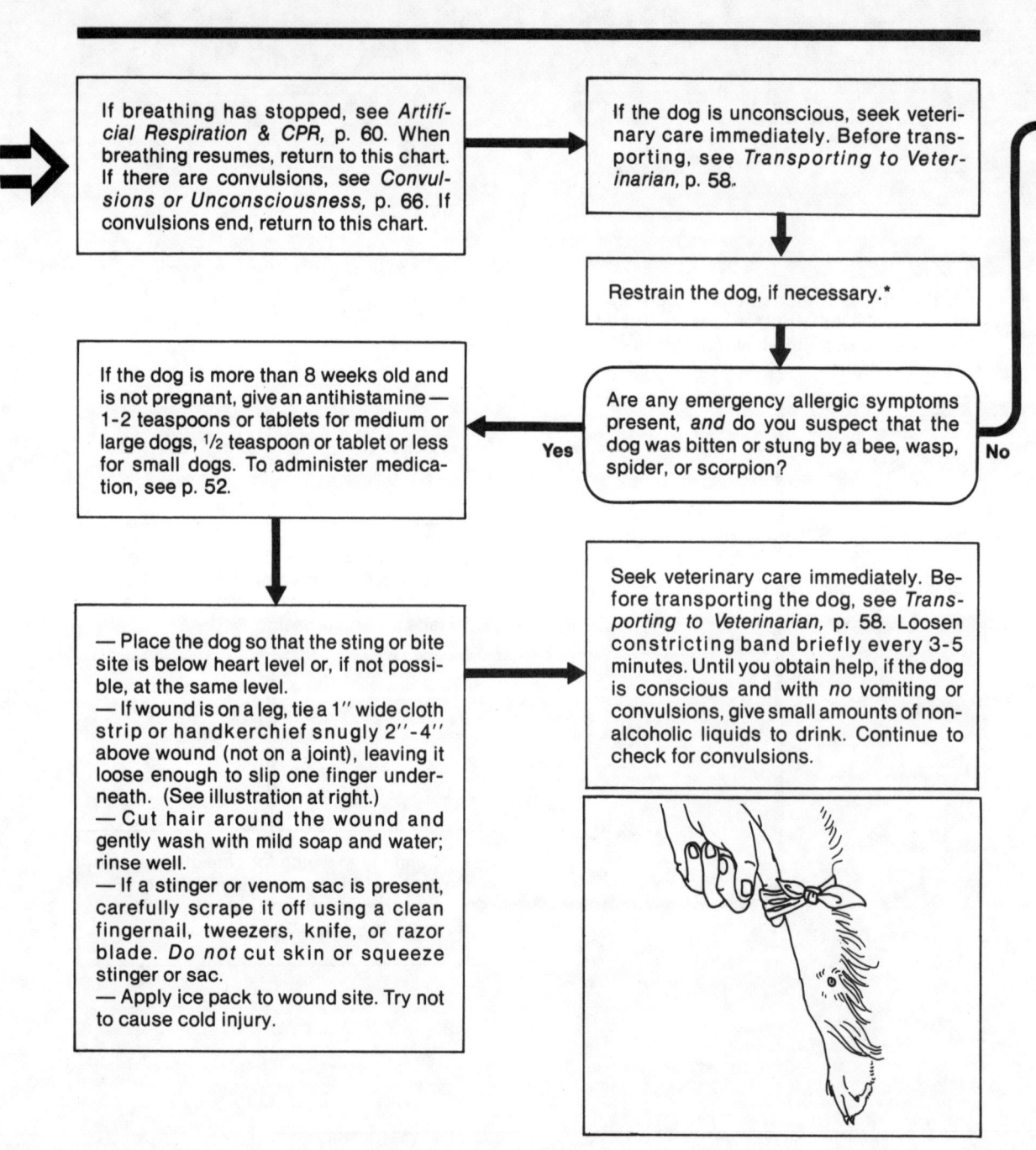

→ If breathing has stopped, see *Artificial Respiration & CPR,* p. 60. When breathing resumes, return to this chart. If there are convulsions, see *Convulsions or Unconsciousness,* p. 66. If convulsions end, return to this chart.

→ If the dog is unconscious, seek veterinary care immediately. Before transporting, see *Transporting to Veterinarian,* p. 58.

↓ Restrain the dog, if necessary.*

↓ Are any emergency allergic symptoms present, *and* do you suspect that the dog was bitten or stung by a bee, wasp, spider, or scorpion?

Yes ← → **No**

If the dog is more than 8 weeks old and is not pregnant, give an antihistamine — 1-2 teaspoons or tablets for medium or large dogs, 1/2 teaspoon or tablet or less for small dogs. To administer medication, see p. 52.

↓

— Place the dog so that the sting or bite site is below heart level or, if not possible, at the same level.
— If wound is on a leg, tie a 1" wide cloth strip or handkerchief snugly 2"-4" above wound (not on a joint), leaving it loose enough to slip one finger underneath. (See illustration at right.)
— Cut hair around the wound and gently wash with mild soap and water; rinse well.
— If a stinger or venom sac is present, carefully scrape it off using a clean fingernail, tweezers, knife, or razor blade. *Do not* cut skin or squeeze stinger or sac.
— Apply ice pack to wound site. Try not to cause cold injury.

Seek veterinary care immediately. Before transporting the dog, see *Transporting to Veterinarian,* p. 58. Loosen constricting band briefly every 3-5 minutes. Until you obtain help, if the dog is conscious and with *no* vomiting or convulsions, give small amounts of non-alcoholic liquids to drink. Continue to check for convulsions.

Possible Signs & Symptoms:
Emergency allergic reaction: *fever/difficult breathing/severe wound/swelling, itching, or pain at bite site/hives/balding or redness/convulsions or loss of consciousness. Blisters and other reactions may not appear for several hours.* **Less serious:** *local irritation or redness/moderate swelling, itching, or pain at bite site.*

Calm the dog by speaking gently.

Are fleas or chiggers (small and dark, or miniscule and reddish, wingless insects) present on the dog's head, back abdomen, ears, or elsewhere?

Yes → If a flea collar is presently being used, remove before applying any of the following treatments, and check with a veterinarian before putting it on again. Apply a flea spray or powder, following package directions carefully. You can use a flea dip instead, but before applying it, ask a veterinarian for directions.

No ↓

Is a tick (a dark, wingless insect) partially embedded in the dog's skin?

Yes →
— Do not crush tick(s) or handle them with your bare hands.
— If 5 or fewer ticks are present, cover each thoroughly with a large amount of petroleum jelly or lip balm.
— If many ticks are present, use a tick spray or powder, following package directions carefully. You can use a tick dip instead, but before applying it, ask a veterinarian for directions.
— After 30 minutes, if tick(s) appear to be easily removable, pull off gently with tweezers; then burn the tick(s) by holding under an open flame.
— Seek veterinary care if ticks are not easily removable.

No ↓

If a stinger or venom sac is present, carefully scrape it off with a clean fingernail, tweezers, knife, or razor blade. *Do not* cut skin or squeeze stinger or sac. Gently wash the wound with mild soap and water and rinse well. If swelling is present, apply cold compresses or a paste of baking soda and water to the site(s). Watch for signs of infection or allergic reaction. If they appear, seek veterinary care immediately.

---

* Restraining Procedure:

Muzzling: Do not muzzle, or if muzzled, remove immediately, if the dog is unconscious, convulsing, vomiting, having difficulty breathing or there is blood or other matter in mouth. For a short-nosed dog, wrap a thick towel firmly around head and neck, securing ends. For a long-nosed dog, bring a long gauze or cloth strip under chin; make a single half-knot on top, bring back under chin, tie a single half-knot again, and bring ends behind head, tying securely with a bow. Do not knot.

Restraining: If the dog is not lying down, straddle his back, facing his head. Gently but firmly hold him with your legs. To have him sit, press on hind quarters; to have him lie, apply firm, gentle pressure gradually to upper back.
— If there are two persons, second person can now treat the dog.
— If you are alone, hold the dog firmly with your legs and one arm, or strap with ties, belts, etc., before treating.

Leg Fractures, Sprains & Dislocations

Do not try to set, straighten, or pop back into place any injured part.

→ Gently restrain the dog, if necessary. (See Restraining Procedure box.) Move him if he is in an unsafe area, keeping his back and neck as straight as possible, and have him lie quietly on his uninjured — or less injured — side.

Restraining Procedure:
Muzzling: * For a short-nosed dog, wrap a thick towel firmly around head and neck, securing ends. For a long-nosed dog, bring a long gauze or cloth strip under chin; make a single half-knot on top, bring back under chin, tie a single half-knot again, and bring ends behind head, tying securely with a bow. Do not knot.
Move the dog if in an unsafe area, keeping his back and neck as straight as possible.
Restraining: If the dog is not lying down, straddle his back, facing his head. Gently but firmly hold him with your legs. To have him sit, press on hind quarters; to have him lie, apply firm, gentle pressure gradually to upper back.
— If there are two persons, second person can now treat the dog.
— If you are alone, hold the dog firmly with your legs and one arm, or strap with ties, belts, etc., before treating.

Has breathing stopped?
- **Yes** → See *Artificial Respiration & CPR,* p. 60. When breathing resumes, return to this chart.
- **No** ↓

If there is bleeding, apply gauze pads and gentle pressure to wound(s). Tape around dressing.

Is there swelling or pain at injured site with *no* other symptoms, such as deformity or protrusion of bones?
- **No** → Do not allow the dog to bear weight on the injured limb for at least another day — until symptoms disappear. Watch for development of other symptoms. If they appear, consult a veterinarian.
- **Yes** ↓

Apply a plastic bag of ice, wrapped in a towel, to the swollen area for 20 minutes every 2 hours. Try to avoid causing cold injury.

→ After 24 hours, is there swelling, or does the dog appear to be suffering as much as before?
- **No** ↑ (return to previous box)
- **Yes** →

Possible Signs & Symptoms: *swelling/ deformity/pain at injured site/sound of bones rubbing together/avoidance of use of limb/protrusion of bone(s).*

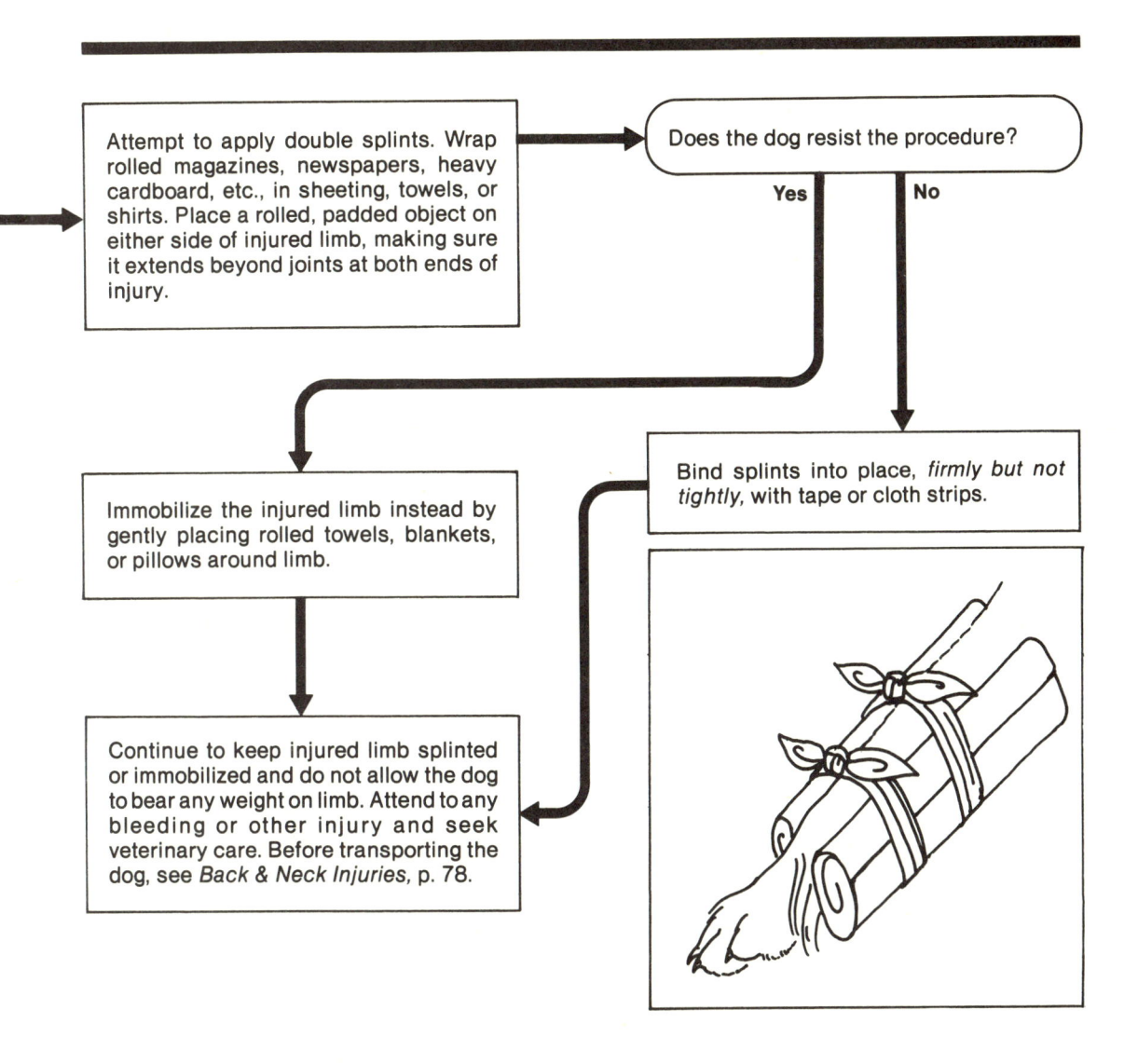

Calm the dog by speaking gently.

Attempt to apply double splints. Wrap rolled magazines, newspapers, heavy cardboard, etc., in sheeting, towels, or shirts. Place a rolled, padded object on either side of injured limb, making sure it extends beyond joints at both ends of injury.

Does the dog resist the procedure?

Yes **No**

Bind splints into place, *firmly but not tightly,* with tape or cloth strips.

Immobilize the injured limb instead by gently placing rolled towels, blankets, or pillows around limb.

Continue to keep injured limb splinted or immobilized and do not allow the dog to bear any weight on limb. Attend to any bleeding or other injury and seek veterinary care. Before transporting the dog, see *Back & Neck Injuries,* p. 78.

*Do not muzzle, or if muzzled, remove immediately, if the dog is unconscious, convulsing, vomiting, having difficulty breathing, or there is blood or other matter in mouth.

Nose Problems
(Including Nosebleed, Foreign Object & Allergy)

If the dog is bleeding from the nose, *and* there is possibly an abdominal, head, or chest injury, see appropriate chart(s): *Abdominal & Chest Injuries*, p. 74, or *Head & Facial Injuries*, p. 86.

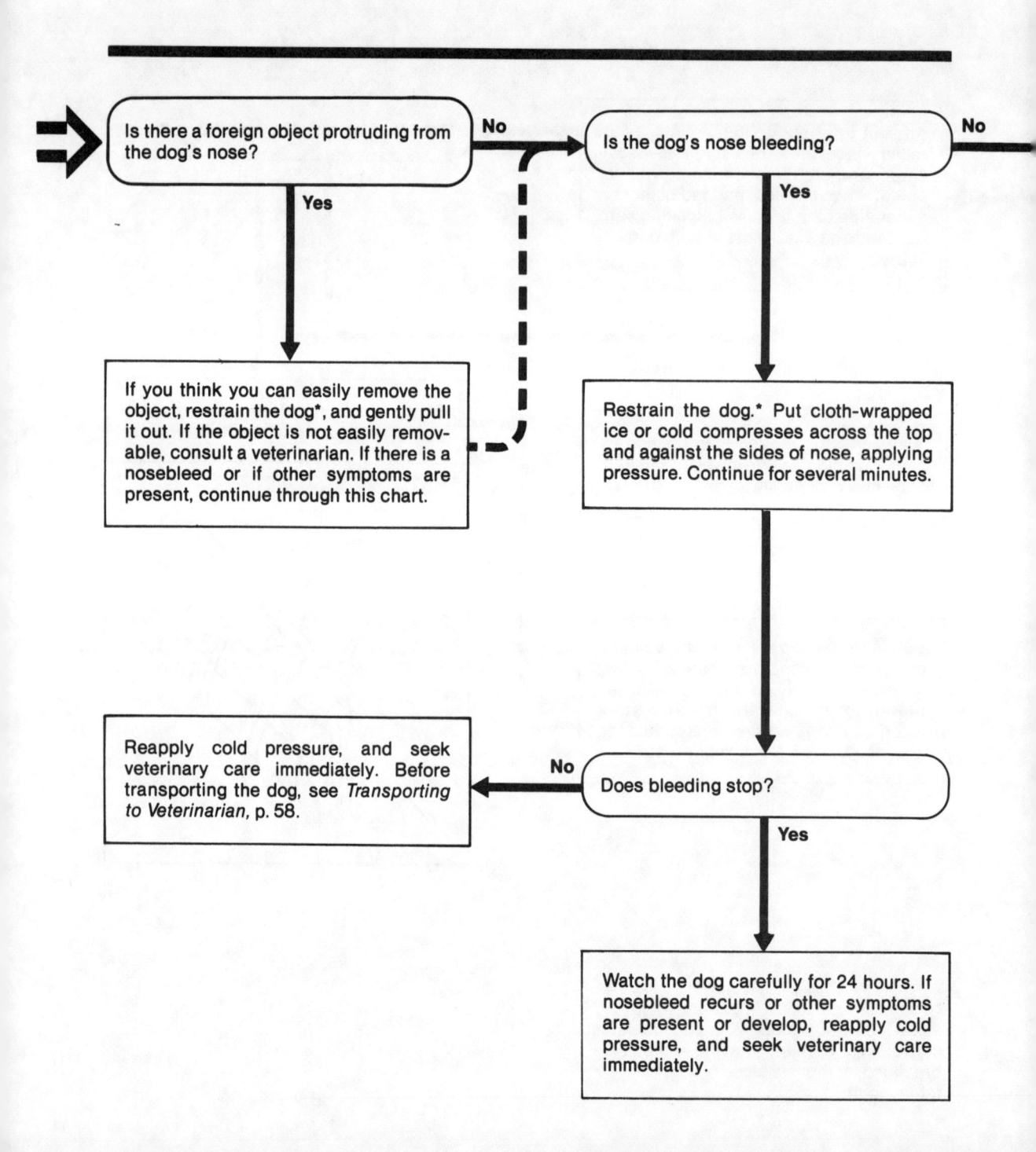

→ **Is there a foreign object protruding from the dog's nose?**

- **No** → **Is the dog's nose bleeding?**
  - **No** →
  - **Yes** ↓

- **Yes** ↓

  If you think you can easily remove the object, restrain the dog*, and gently pull it out. If the object is not easily removable, consult a veterinarian. If there is a nosebleed or if other symptoms are present, continue through this chart.

Restrain the dog.* Put cloth-wrapped ice or cold compresses across the top and against the sides of nose, applying pressure. Continue for several minutes.

↓

Does bleeding stop?

- **No** → Reapply cold pressure, and seek veterinary care immediately. Before transporting the dog, see *Transporting to Veterinarian*, p. 58.
- **Yes** ↓

Watch the dog carefully for 24 hours. If nosebleed recurs or other symptoms are present or develop, reapply cold pressure, and seek veterinary care immediately.

Calm the dog by speaking gently.

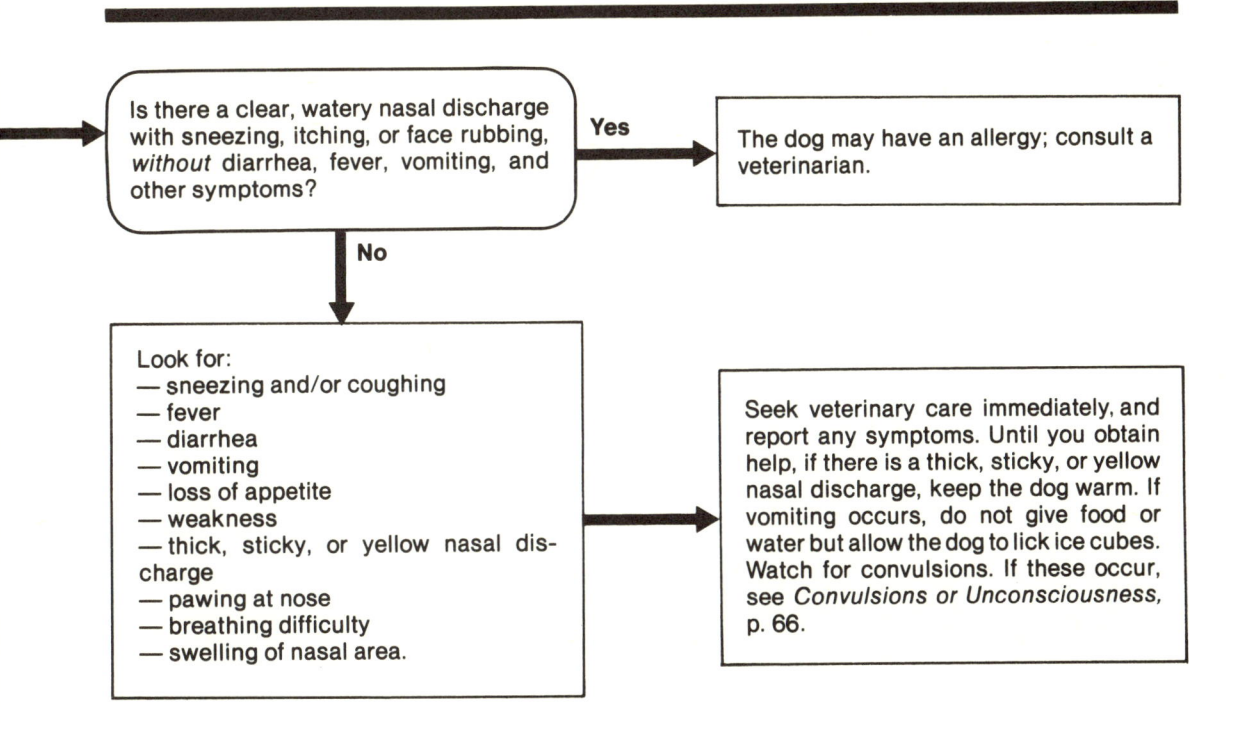

Is there a clear, watery nasal discharge with sneezing, itching, or face rubbing, *without* diarrhea, fever, vomiting, and other symptoms? — **Yes** → The dog may have an allergy; consult a veterinarian.

No ↓

Look for:
— sneezing and/or coughing
— fever
— diarrhea
— vomiting
— loss of appetite
— weakness
— thick, sticky, or yellow nasal discharge
— pawing at nose
— breathing difficulty
— swelling of nasal area.

→ Seek veterinary care immediately, and report any symptoms. Until you obtain help, if there is a thick, sticky, or yellow nasal discharge, keep the dog warm. If vomiting occurs, do not give food or water but allow the dog to lick ice cubes. Watch for convulsions. If these occur, see *Convulsions or Unconsciousness*, p. 66.

* Restraining Procedure:

Muzzling: Do not muzzle, or if muzzled, remove immediately, if the dog is unconscious, convulsing, vomiting, having difficulty breathing or there is blood or other matter in mouth. For a short-nosed dog, wrap a thick towel firmly around head and neck, securing ends. For a long-nosed dog, bring a long gauze or cloth strip under chin; make a single half-knot on top, bring back under chin, tie a single half-knot again, and bring ends behind head, tying securely with a bow. Do not knot.

Restraining: If the dog is not lying down, straddle his back, facing his head. Gently but firmly hold him with your legs. To have him sit, press on hind quarters; to have him lie, apply firm, gentle pressure gradually to upper back.
— If there are two persons, second person can now treat the dog.
— If you are alone, hold the dog firmly with your legs and one arm, or strap with ties, belts, etc., before treating.

Poisoning
(Ingested or Inhaled)

— If you suspect an allergic reaction to an ingested or inhaled substance, see *Allergic Reaction*, p. 76. Symptoms may include swelling, itching, and/or hives.
— For the treatment of burns on the dog's mouth or body, see *Burns*, p. 80.

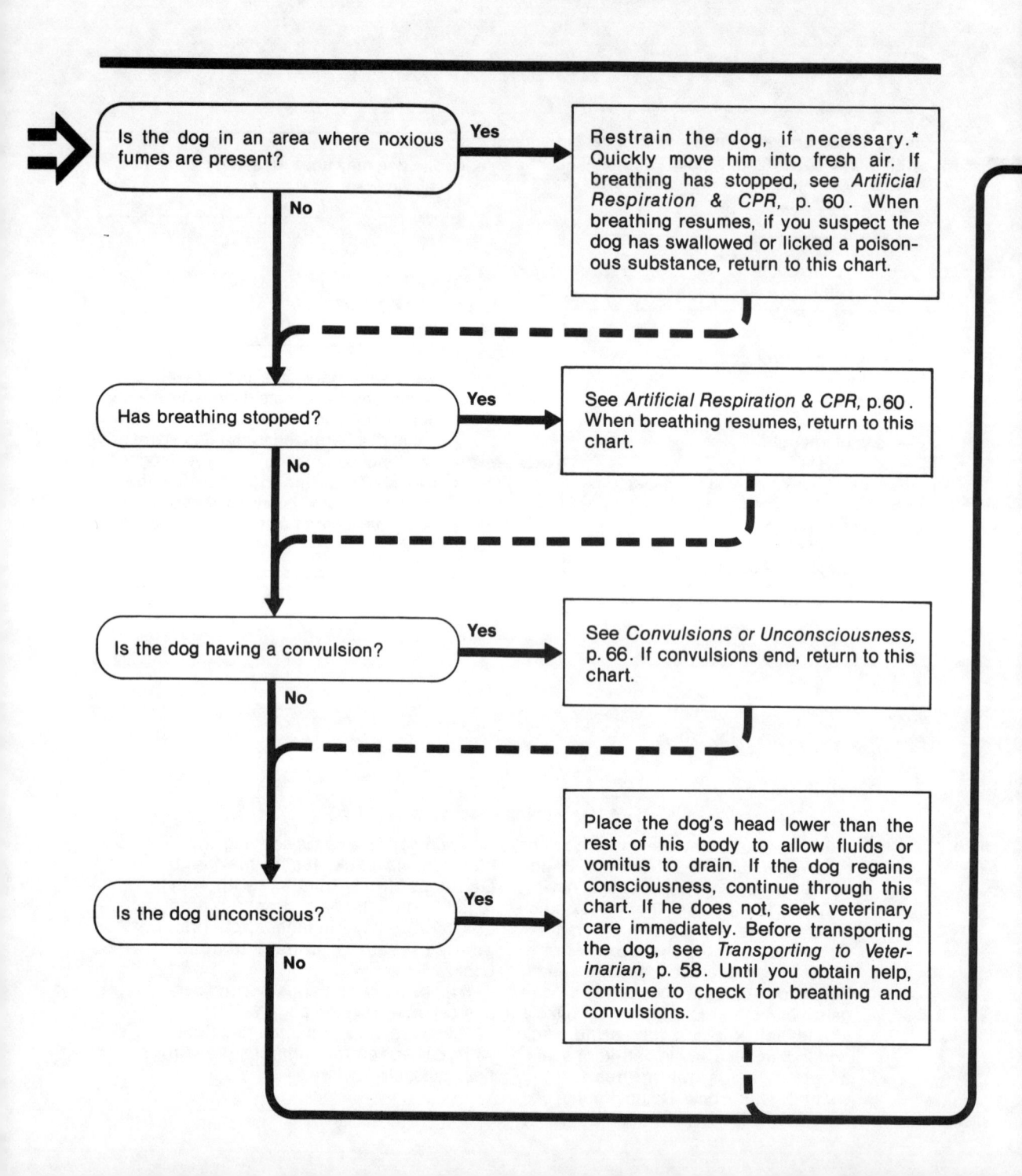

Is the dog in an area where noxious fumes are present?
- **Yes** → Restrain the dog, if necessary.* Quickly move him into fresh air. If breathing has stopped, see *Artificial Respiration & CPR*, p. 60. When breathing resumes, if you suspect the dog has swallowed or licked a poisonous substance, return to this chart.
- **No** ↓

Has breathing stopped?
- **Yes** → See *Artificial Respiration & CPR*, p. 60. When breathing resumes, return to this chart.
- **No** ↓

Is the dog having a convulsion?
- **Yes** → See *Convulsions or Unconsciousness*, p. 66. If convulsions end, return to this chart.
- **No** ↓

Is the dog unconscious?
- **Yes** → Place the dog's head lower than the rest of his body to allow fluids or vomitus to drain. If the dog regains consciousness, continue through this chart. If he does not, seek veterinary care immediately. Before transporting the dog, see *Transporting to Veterinarian*, p. 58. Until you obtain help, continue to check for breathing and convulsions.
- **No** ↓

Possible Signs & Symptoms: *vomiting/diarrhea/painful abdominal area/burns in or around mouth or on other parts of body/difficult breathing/profuse drooling/muscle spasms/weakness/acid odor of vomitus or breath/obvious toxic substance in dog's mouth/convulsions or loss of consciousness/spilled or open container of a toxic substance.*

Calm the dog by speaking gently.

Are there burns in or on the dog's mouth, or is there bloody vomitus or an acid odor on his breath?

Yes → After any vomiting has stopped, remove any restraints and flush mouth out with water. If the dog is without breathing problems or convulsions, give milk, vegetable oil, egg whites, or water to drink.

No ↓

If you suspect the dog has ingested a toxic substance and he is without breathing difficulty or convulsions, remove any restraints and induce vomiting:
— Give syrup of ipecac — dosages are 2-3 teaspoons for medium or large dogs, 1½ teaspoons or less for small dogs and puppies. To administer medication, see p. 52.
— Repeat every 10 minutes up to ½ hour until the dog vomits.
— Save a sample of the vomitus for later evaluation.

↓

After any vomiting subsides, if the dog is still conscious and without convulsions or breathing difficulty, give water or milk mixed with activated charcoal. (See package directions for proper amount.)

→ Seek veterinary care immediately, bringing the vomitus sample or container from which the dog ingested the toxic substance, if available. Before transporting the dog, see *Transporting to Veterinarian,* p. 58. Until you obtain help, watch for choking and convulsions. Attend to any burns. (See *Burns,* p. 80.)

* Restraining Procedure:
Muzzling: Do not muzzle, or if muzzled, remove immediately, if the dog is unconscious, convulsing, vomiting, having difficulty breathing, or there is blood or other matter in mouth. For a short-nosed dog, wrap a thick towel firmly around head and neck, securing ends. For a long-nosed dog, bring a long gauze or cloth strip under chin; make a single half-knot on top, bring back under chin, tie a single half-knot again, and bring ends behind head, tying securely with a bow. Do not knot. Move the dog if in an unsafe area.

Snakebite

Follow these procedures *immediately* after snakebite.

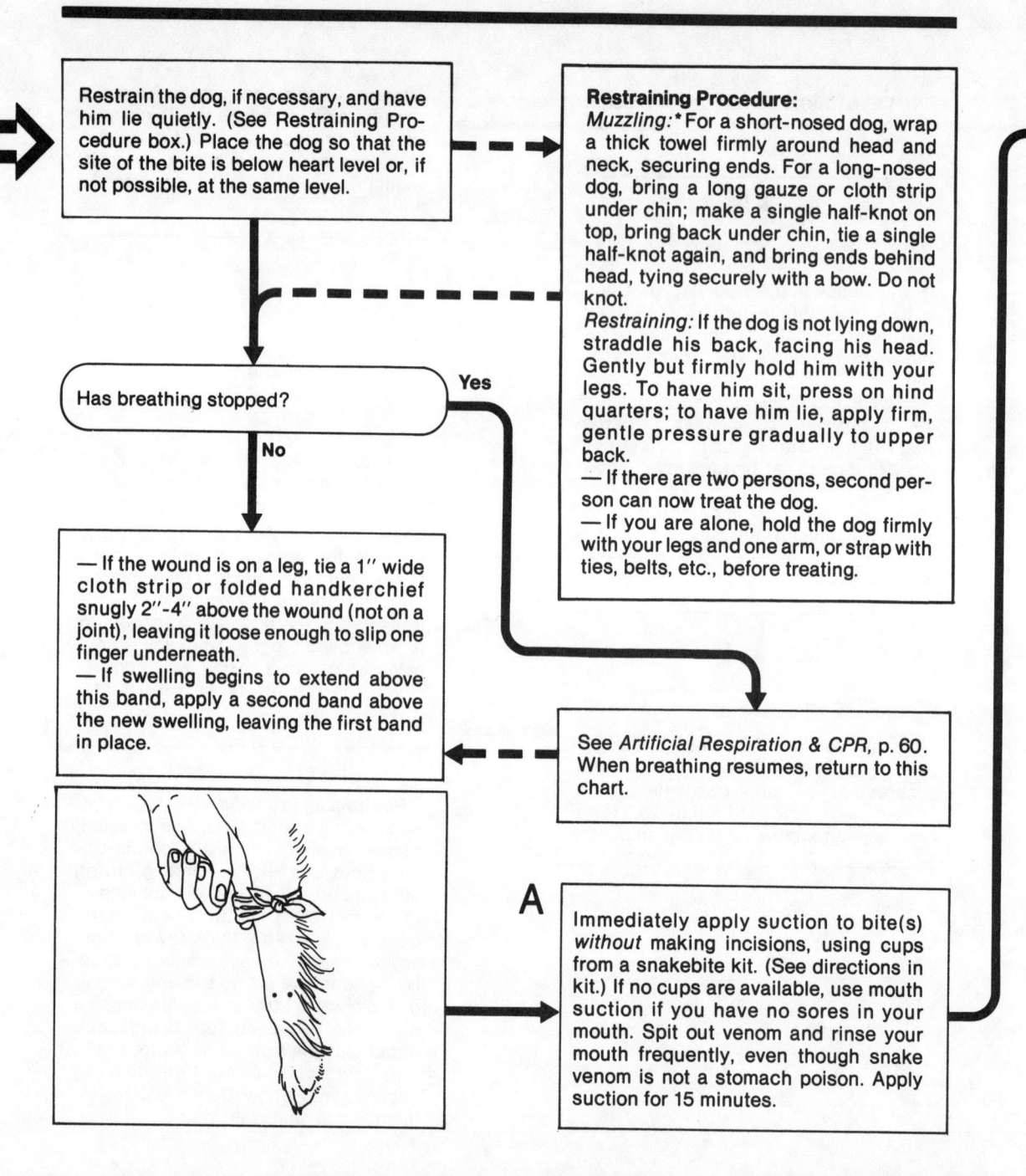

→ Restrain the dog, if necessary, and have him lie quietly. (See Restraining Procedure box.) Place the dog so that the site of the bite is below heart level or, if not possible, at the same level.

Restraining Procedure:
Muzzling: *For a short-nosed dog, wrap a thick towel firmly around head and neck, securing ends. For a long-nosed dog, bring a long gauze or cloth strip under chin; make a single half-knot on top, bring back under chin, tie a single half-knot again, and bring ends behind head, tying securely with a bow. Do not knot.
Restraining: If the dog is not lying down, straddle his back, facing his head. Gently but firmly hold him with your legs. To have him sit, press on hind quarters; to have him lie, apply firm, gentle pressure gradually to upper back.
— If there are two persons, second person can now treat the dog.
— If you are alone, hold the dog firmly with your legs and one arm, or strap with ties, belts, etc., before treating.

Has breathing stopped?

Yes → See *Artificial Respiration & CPR*, p. 60. When breathing resumes, return to this chart.

No ↓

— If the wound is on a leg, tie a 1" wide cloth strip or folded handkerchief snugly 2"-4" above the wound (not on a joint), leaving it loose enough to slip one finger underneath.
— If swelling begins to extend above this band, apply a second band above the new swelling, leaving the first band in place.

A Immediately apply suction to bite(s) *without* making incisions, using cups from a snakebite kit. (See directions in kit.) If no cups are available, use mouth suction if you have no sores in your mouth. Spit out venom and rinse your mouth frequently, even though snake venom is not a stomach poison. Apply suction for 15 minutes.

Possible Signs & Symptoms
Poisonous: 1–2 fang marks, commonly found on face or legs / severe swelling and pain at wound site / weakness / vomiting / difficult breathing / convulsions or loss of consciousness. Coral snake reactions, though poisonous, may appear less severe and be delayed up to 18 hours.

Calm the dog by speaking gently.

After suctioning for 15 minutes, is there swelling or pain at the wound site? — **No** → Unless the wound was caused by a coral snake, either the snake was not poisonous, or little or no venom was absorbed. Cut the hair around the wound and wash the wound with soap and water or rubbing alcohol. Apply cold, wet compresses.

Yes ↓

Will the dog receive medical assistance within 60 minutes of having been bitten?
OR
Was he bitten by a coral snake? — **Yes** → Continue to check the bite area, and seek veterinary care immediately, even if you assume the bite was not poisonous. Watch for convulsions. If these occur, see *Convulsions or Unconsciousness,* p. 66. Remove constricting bands after 1–2 hours. If the dog is conscious and not vomiting or convulsing, remove any restraints and give small amounts of nonalcoholic liquids to drink. Before transporting the dog, see *Transporting to Veterinarian,* p. 58.

No ↓

— Cut the hair around the wound and wash the wound with soap and water or rubbing alcohol.
— Sterilize a knife or razor blade with rubbing alcohol or by holding under an open flame.
— Make a linear — not crosswise — incision through each fang mark, about 1/4" long and not more than 1/8" deep. *Do not* cut through a vein.

punctures
incisions

Again, apply suction as directed in Box A. If snakebite kit containing antivenin is available, use as directed in package, and be sure to test for allergy as instructed. Leave band(s) in place, wash the wound again, and apply cold, wet compresses.

*Do not muzzle, or if muzzled, remove immediately, if the dog is unconscious, convulsing, vomiting, having difficulty breathing, or there is blood or other matter in mouth.

Swelling

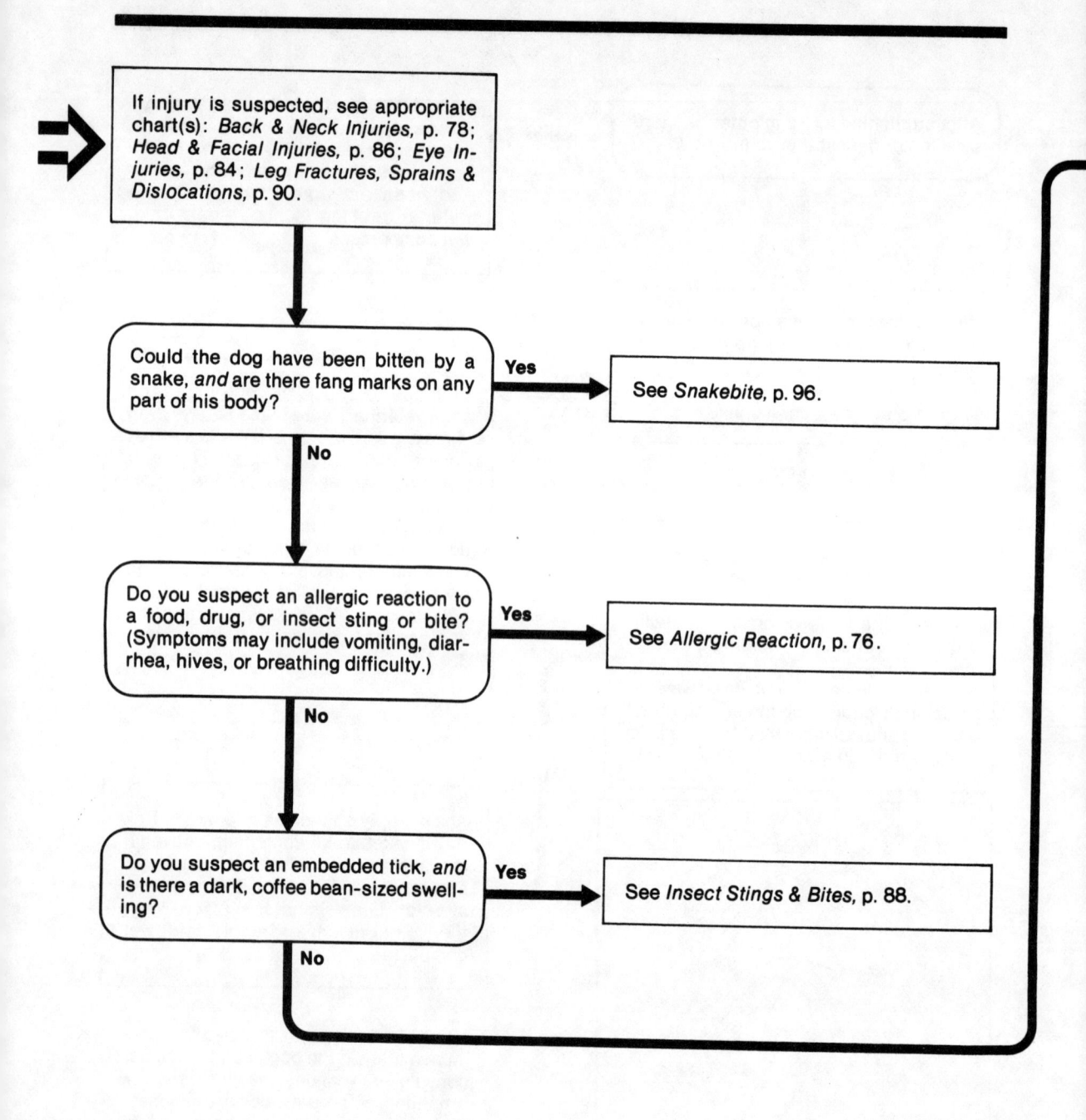

→ If injury is suspected, see appropriate chart(s): *Back & Neck Injuries*, p. 78; *Head & Facial Injuries*, p. 86; *Eye Injuries*, p. 84; *Leg Fractures, Sprains & Dislocations*, p. 90.

↓

Could the dog have been bitten by a snake, *and* are there fang marks on any part of his body? —**Yes**→ See *Snakebite*, p. 96.

↓ **No**

Do you suspect an allergic reaction to a food, drug, or insect sting or bite? (Symptoms may include vomiting, diarrhea, hives, or breathing difficulty.) —**Yes**→ See *Allergic Reaction*, p. 76.

↓ **No**

Do you suspect an embedded tick, *and* is there a dark, coffee bean-sized swelling? —**Yes**→ See *Insect Stings & Bites*, p. 88.

↓ **No**

Calm the dog by speaking gently.

→ Is the dog a female who has been weaning, *and* is there swelling of the mammary gland and/or glands with no hardness or pain, *and* does the dog seem otherwise healthy? —**Yes**→ Place cold compresses on the affected gland and/or glands for 15 minutes, three times a day. If swelling persists for more than 2 days, seek veterinary care.

↓ **No**

Is the swollen area between the dog's toes? —**Yes**→ Restrain the dog, if necessary. (See Restraining Procedure box.) Check area for the presence of a foreign object; remove it if visible and within reach. Wash area well with mild soap and water, rinse well, and apply an antibiotic ointment. If swelling is severe or persists more than 2 days or if other symptoms develop, contact a veterinarian.

↓ **No**

Look for:
— pain
— pus
— fever
— redness
— hardness
— severe swelling of abdomen or chest
— vomiting
— loss of appetite
— anxiety or depression
— diarrhea
— strained passage of feces or urine
— swelling in groin or, in male dogs, the scrotum
— breathing difficulty.

↓

Seek veterinary care immediately, and report any symptoms. Until you obtain help, keep the dog comfortable and quiet. If the dog appears very ill, see *Transporting to Veterinarian,* p. 58, before transporting.

Restraining Procedure:
Muzzling:* For a short-nosed dog, wrap a thick towel firmly around head and neck, securing ends. For a long-nosed dog, bring a long gauze or cloth strip under chin; make a single half-knot on top, bring back under chin, tie a single half-knot again, and bring ends behind head, tying securely with a bow. Do not knot.
Restraining: If the dog is not lying down, straddle his back, facing his head. Gently but firmly hold him with your legs. To have him sit, press on hind quarters; to have him lie, apply firm, gentle pressure gradually to upper back.
— If there are two persons, second person can now treat the dog.
— If you are alone, hold the dog firmly with your legs and one arm, or strap with ties, belts, etc., before treating.

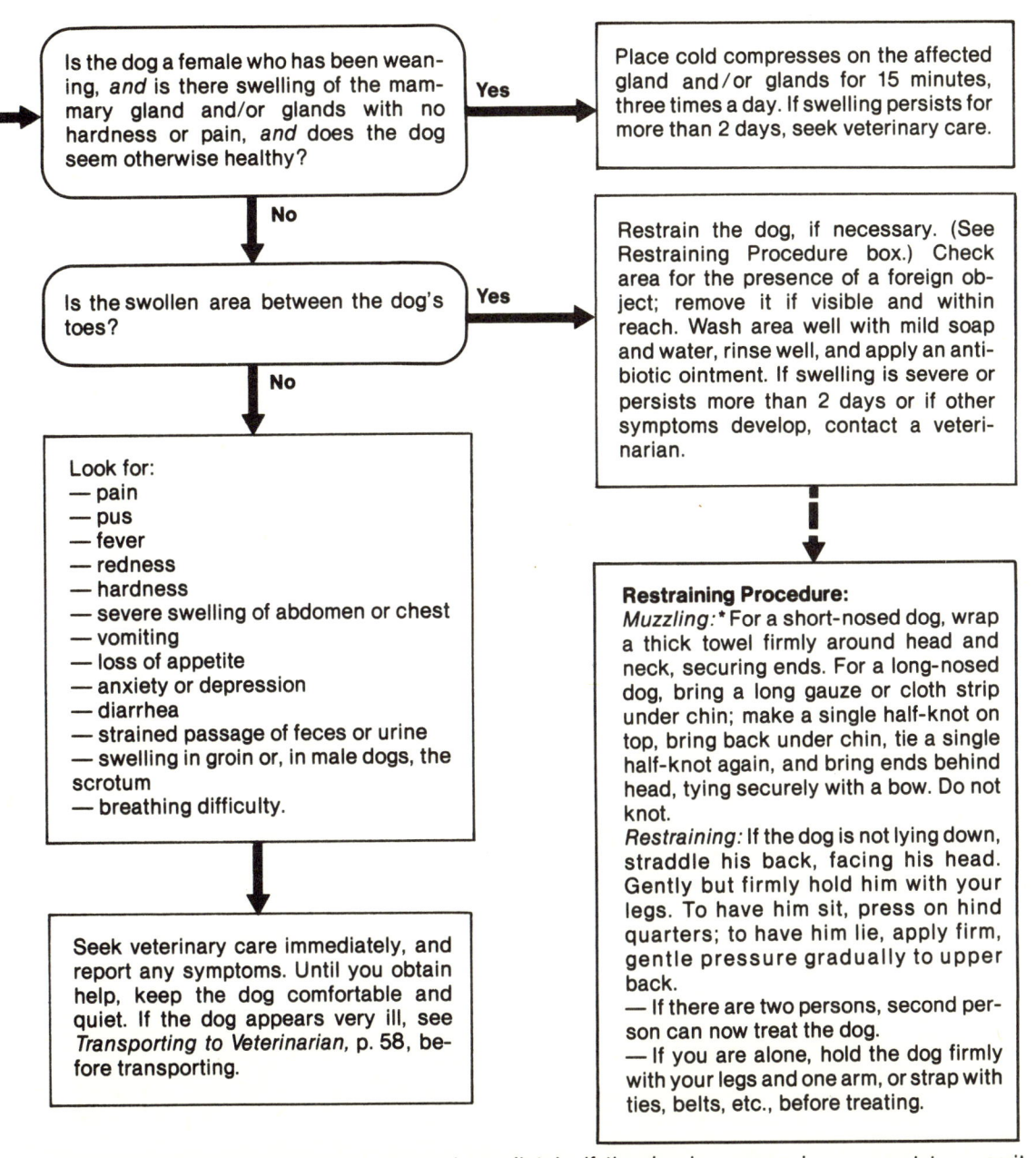

*Do not muzzle, or if muzzled, remove immediately, if the dog is unconscious, convulsing, vomiting, having difficulty breathing, or there is blood or other matter in mouth.

Tooth & Mouth Injuries
(Including Burns & Foreign Object)

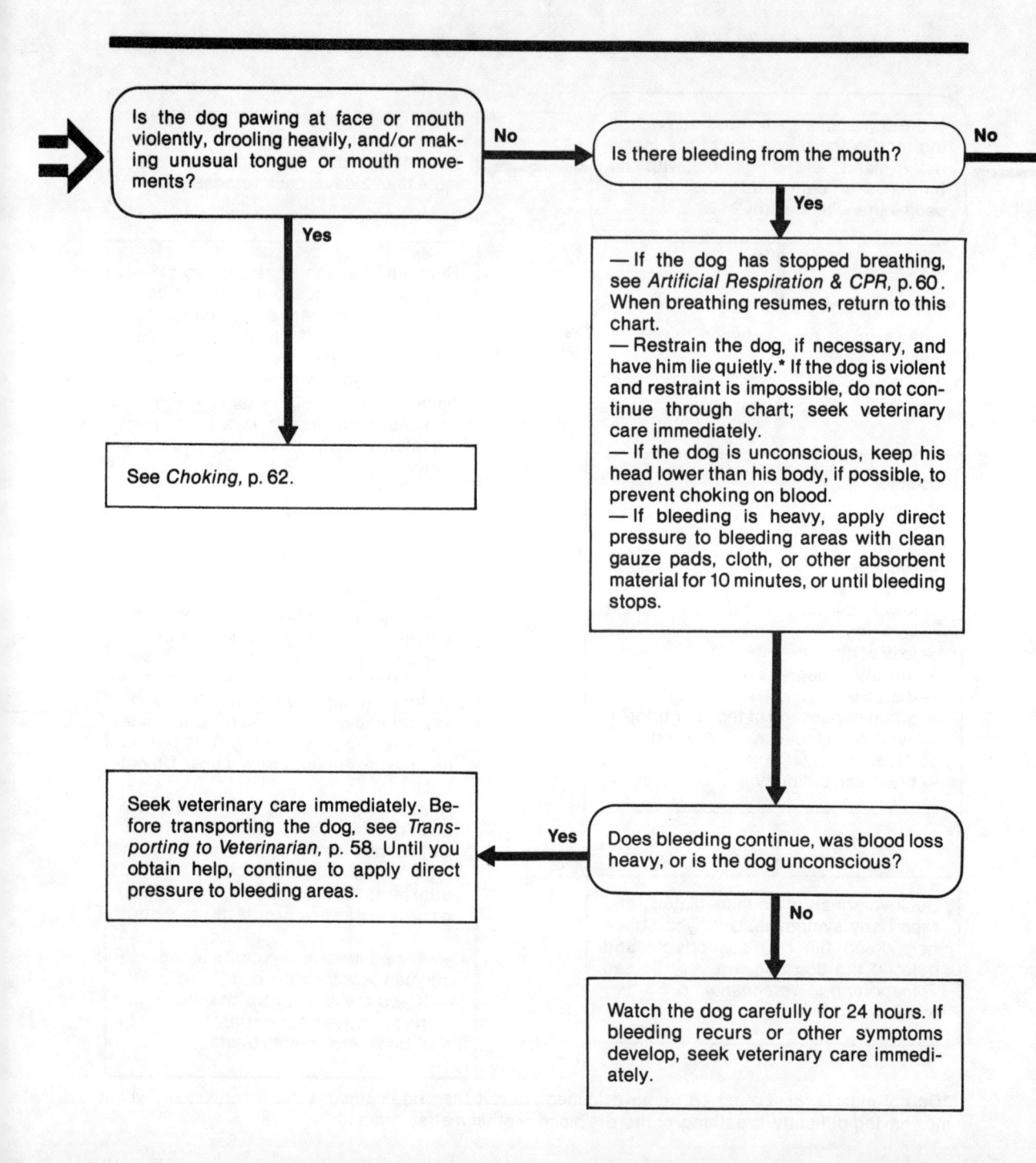

→ Is the dog pawing at face or mouth violently, drooling heavily, and/or making unusual tongue or mouth movements?

- **Yes** → See *Choking*, p. 62.
- **No** → Is there bleeding from the mouth?
  - **No** →
  - **Yes** →
    - If the dog has stopped breathing, see *Artificial Respiration & CPR*, p. 60. When breathing resumes, return to this chart.
    - Restrain the dog, if necessary, and have him lie quietly.* If the dog is violent and restraint is impossible, do not continue through chart; seek veterinary care immediately.
    - If the dog is unconscious, keep his head lower than his body, if possible, to prevent choking on blood.
    - If bleeding is heavy, apply direct pressure to bleeding areas with clean gauze pads, cloth, or other absorbent material for 10 minutes, or until bleeding stops.

Does bleeding continue, was blood loss heavy, or is the dog unconscious?

- **Yes** → Seek veterinary care immediately. Before transporting the dog, see *Transporting to Veterinarian*, p. 58. Until you obtain help, continue to apply direct pressure to bleeding areas.
- **No** → Watch the dog carefully for 24 hours. If bleeding recurs or other symptoms develop, seek veterinary care immediately.

If the dog is bleeding from the mouth, *and* **there is possibly an abdominal, head, or chest injury, see appropriate chart(s):** *Abdominal & Chest Injuries,* **p. 74, or** *Head & Facial Injuries,* **p. 86.**

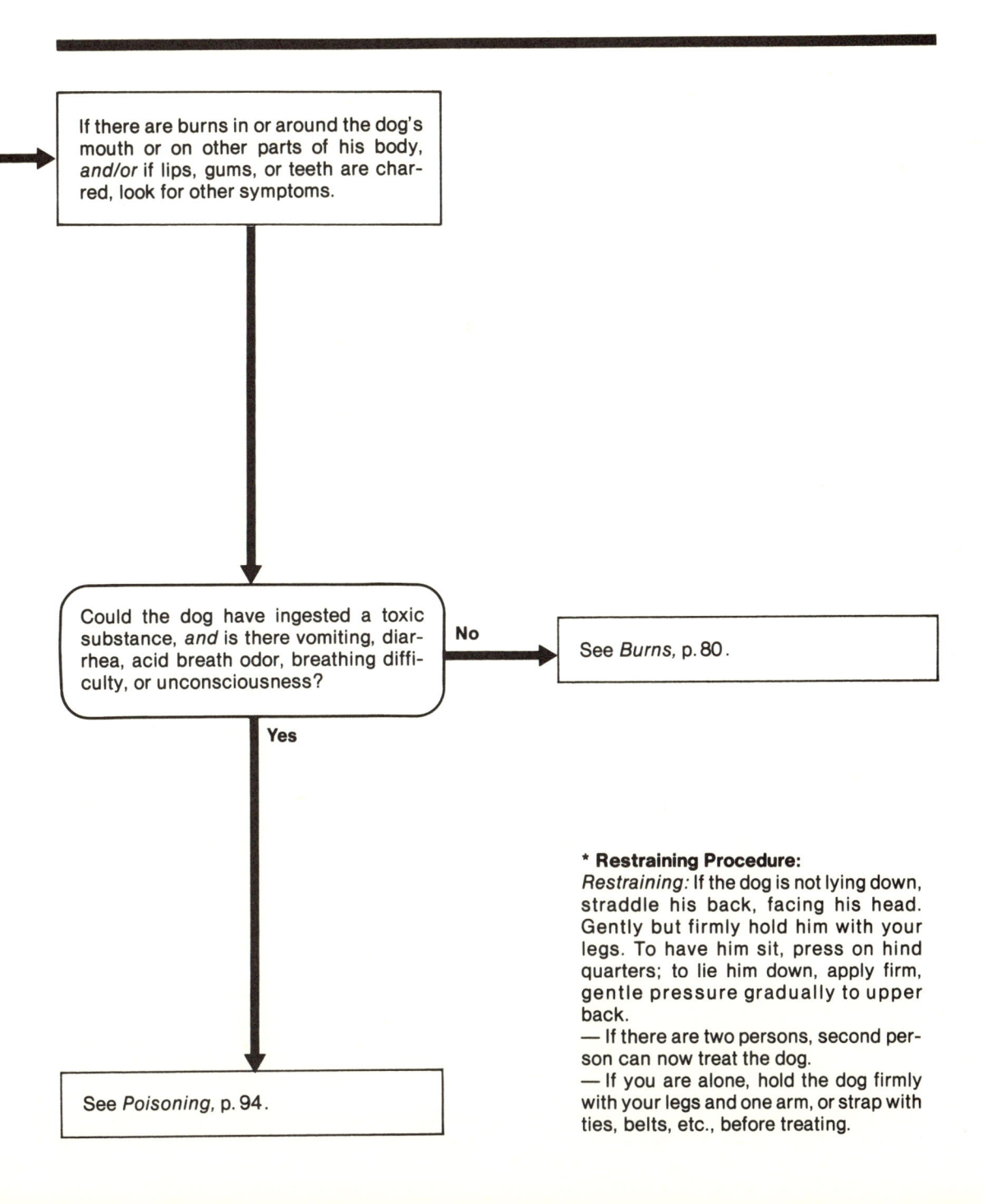

Calm the dog by speaking gently.

If there are burns in or around the dog's mouth or on other parts of his body, *and/or* if lips, gums, or teeth are charred, look for other symptoms.

↓

Could the dog have ingested a toxic substance, *and* is there vomiting, diarrhea, acid breath odor, breathing difficulty, or unconsciousness? — **No** → See *Burns,* p. 80.

Yes ↓

See *Poisoning,* p. 94.

* Restraining Procedure:
Restraining: If the dog is not lying down, straddle his back, facing his head. Gently but firmly hold him with your legs. To have him sit, press on hind quarters; to lie him down, apply firm, gentle pressure gradually to upper back.
— If there are two persons, second person can now treat the dog.
— If you are alone, hold the dog firmly with your legs and one arm, or strap with ties, belts, etc., before treating.

Puncture & Deep Wounds
(Including Major Animal Bites)

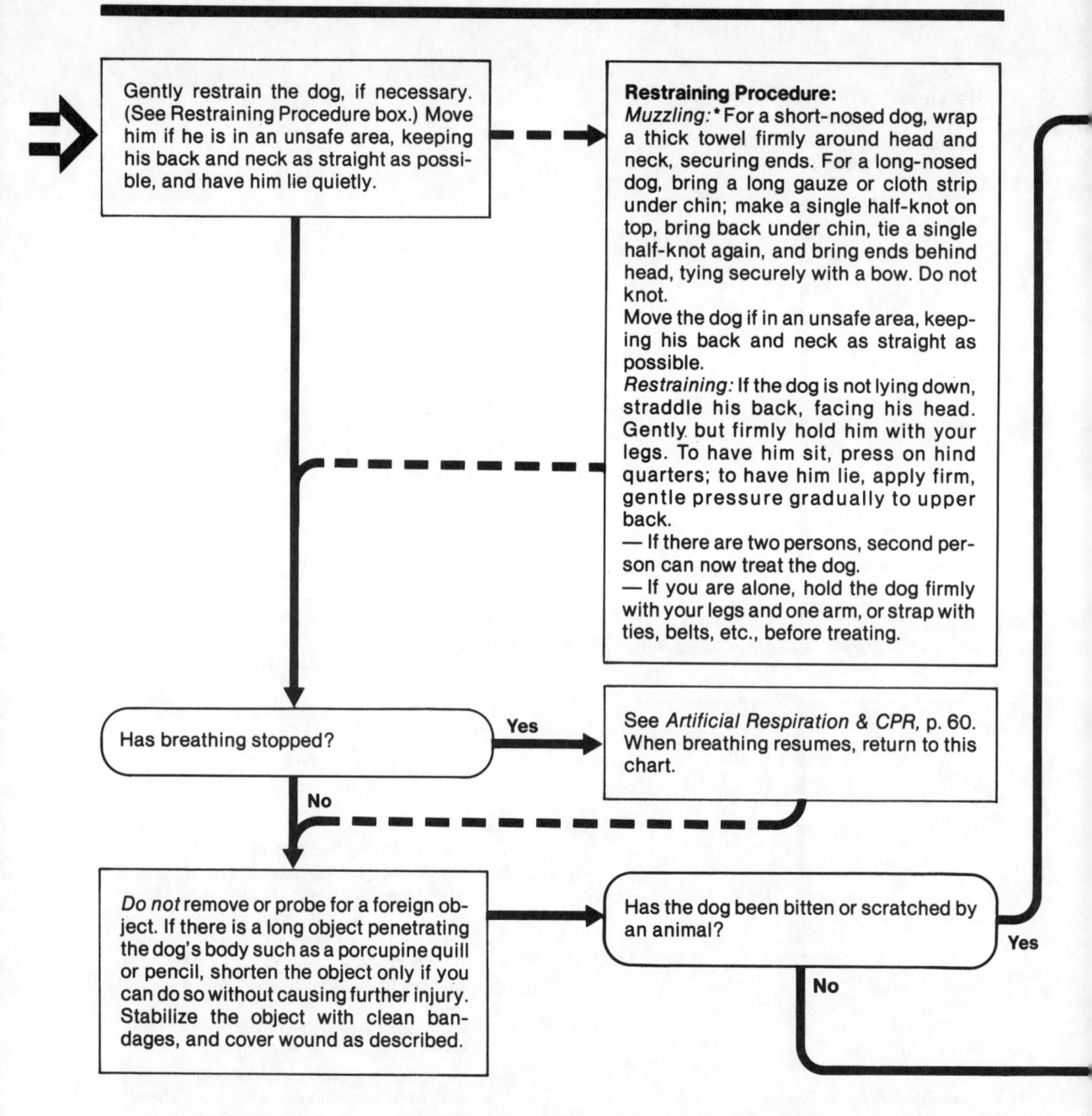

→ Gently restrain the dog, if necessary. (See Restraining Procedure box.) Move him if he is in an unsafe area, keeping his back and neck as straight as possible, and have him lie quietly.

Restraining Procedure:
Muzzling:* For a short-nosed dog, wrap a thick towel firmly around head and neck, securing ends. For a long-nosed dog, bring a long gauze or cloth strip under chin; make a single half-knot on top, bring back under chin, tie a single half-knot again, and bring ends behind head, tying securely with a bow. Do not knot.
Move the dog if in an unsafe area, keeping his back and neck as straight as possible.
Restraining: If the dog is not lying down, straddle his back, facing his head. Gently but firmly hold him with your legs. To have him sit, press on hind quarters; to have him lie, apply firm, gentle pressure gradually to upper back.
— If there are two persons, second person can now treat the dog.
— If you are alone, hold the dog firmly with your legs and one arm, or strap with ties, belts, etc., before treating.

Has breathing stopped? — **Yes** → See *Artificial Respiration & CPR,* p. 60. When breathing resumes, return to this chart.

No ↓

Do not remove or probe for a foreign object. If there is a long object penetrating the dog's body such as a porcupine quill or pencil, shorten the object only if you can do so without causing further injury. Stabilize the object with clean bandages, and cover wound as described.

Has the dog been bitten or scratched by an animal? — **Yes** / **No**

---

*Do not muzzle, or if muzzled, remove immediately, if the dog is unconscious, convulsing, vomiting, having difficulty breathing, or there is blood or other matter in mouth.

For eye injuries, see p. 84; *for abdominal or chest wounds,* see p. 74; *for head wounds,* see p. 86. If the dog may have been bitten by a snake, see p. 96.

Do not attempt to set, straighten, or pop back into place any injured part.

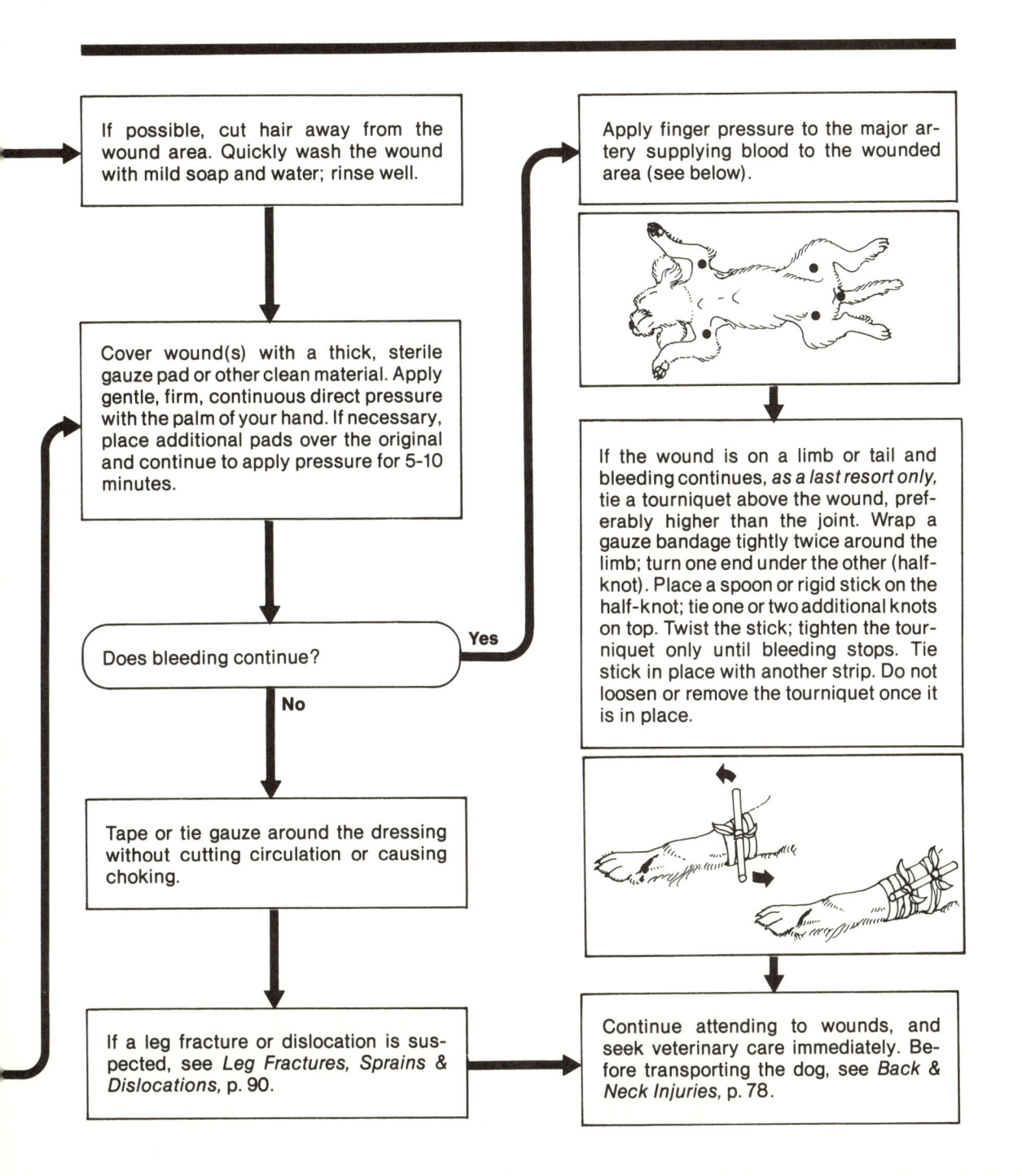

Calm the dog by speaking gently.

If possible, cut hair away from the wound area. Quickly wash the wound with mild soap and water; rinse well.

Cover wound(s) with a thick, sterile gauze pad or other clean material. Apply gentle, firm, continuous direct pressure with the palm of your hand. If necessary, place additional pads over the original and continue to apply pressure for 5-10 minutes.

Does bleeding continue?

No → Tape or tie gauze around the dressing without cutting circulation or causing choking.

If a leg fracture or dislocation is suspected, see *Leg Fractures, Sprains & Dislocations,* p. 90.

Yes → Apply finger pressure to the major artery supplying blood to the wounded area (see below).

If the wound is on a limb or tail and bleeding continues, *as a last resort only,* tie a tourniquet above the wound, preferably higher than the joint. Wrap a gauze bandage tightly twice around the limb; turn one end under the other (half-knot). Place a spoon or rigid stick on the half-knot; tie one or two additional knots on top. Twist the stick; tighten the tourniquet only until bleeding stops. Tie stick in place with another strip. Do not loosen or remove the tourniquet once it is in place.

Continue attending to wounds, and seek veterinary care immediately. Before transporting the dog, see *Back & Neck Injuries,* p. 78.

Cold Exposure & Frostbite

To take the dog's temperature, see p. 51.

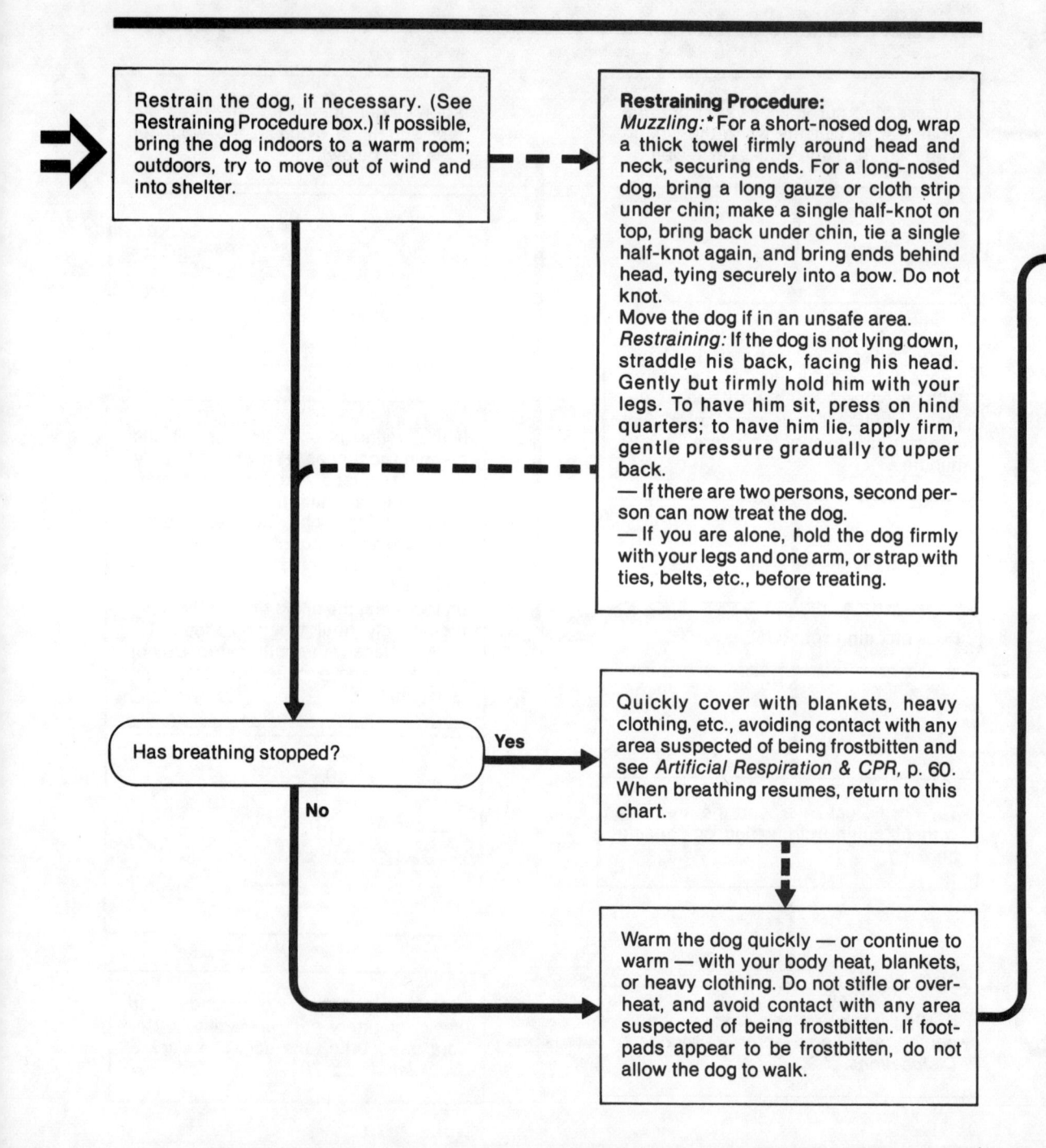

→ Restrain the dog, if necessary. (See Restraining Procedure box.) If possible, bring the dog indoors to a warm room; outdoors, try to move out of wind and into shelter.

Restraining Procedure:
*Muzzling:** For a short-nosed dog, wrap a thick towel firmly around head and neck, securing ends. For a long-nosed dog, bring a long gauze or cloth strip under chin; make a single half-knot on top, bring back under chin, tie a single half-knot again, and bring ends behind head, tying securely into a bow. Do not knot.
Move the dog if in an unsafe area.
Restraining: If the dog is not lying down, straddle his back, facing his head. Gently but firmly hold him with your legs. To have him sit, press on hind quarters; to have him lie, apply firm, gentle pressure gradually to upper back.
— If there are two persons, second person can now treat the dog.
— If you are alone, hold the dog firmly with your legs and one arm, or strap with ties, belts, etc., before treating.

Has breathing stopped?

Yes → Quickly cover with blankets, heavy clothing, etc., avoiding contact with any area suspected of being frostbitten and see *Artificial Respiration & CPR*, p. 60. When breathing resumes, return to this chart.

No ↓

Warm the dog quickly — or continue to warm — with your body heat, blankets, or heavy clothing. Do not stifle or overheat, and avoid contact with any area suspected of being frostbitten. If footpads appear to be frostbitten, do not allow the dog to walk.

Possible Signs & Symptoms
Cold Exposure (Hypothermia): *temperature of 90°F or less/shivering/drowsiness/difficulty walking/loss of consciousness.*
Frostbite: *pale, stiff, or red and scaly areas not protected by hair such as foot pads, ear tips, and scrotum/pain at affected areas in early stages.*

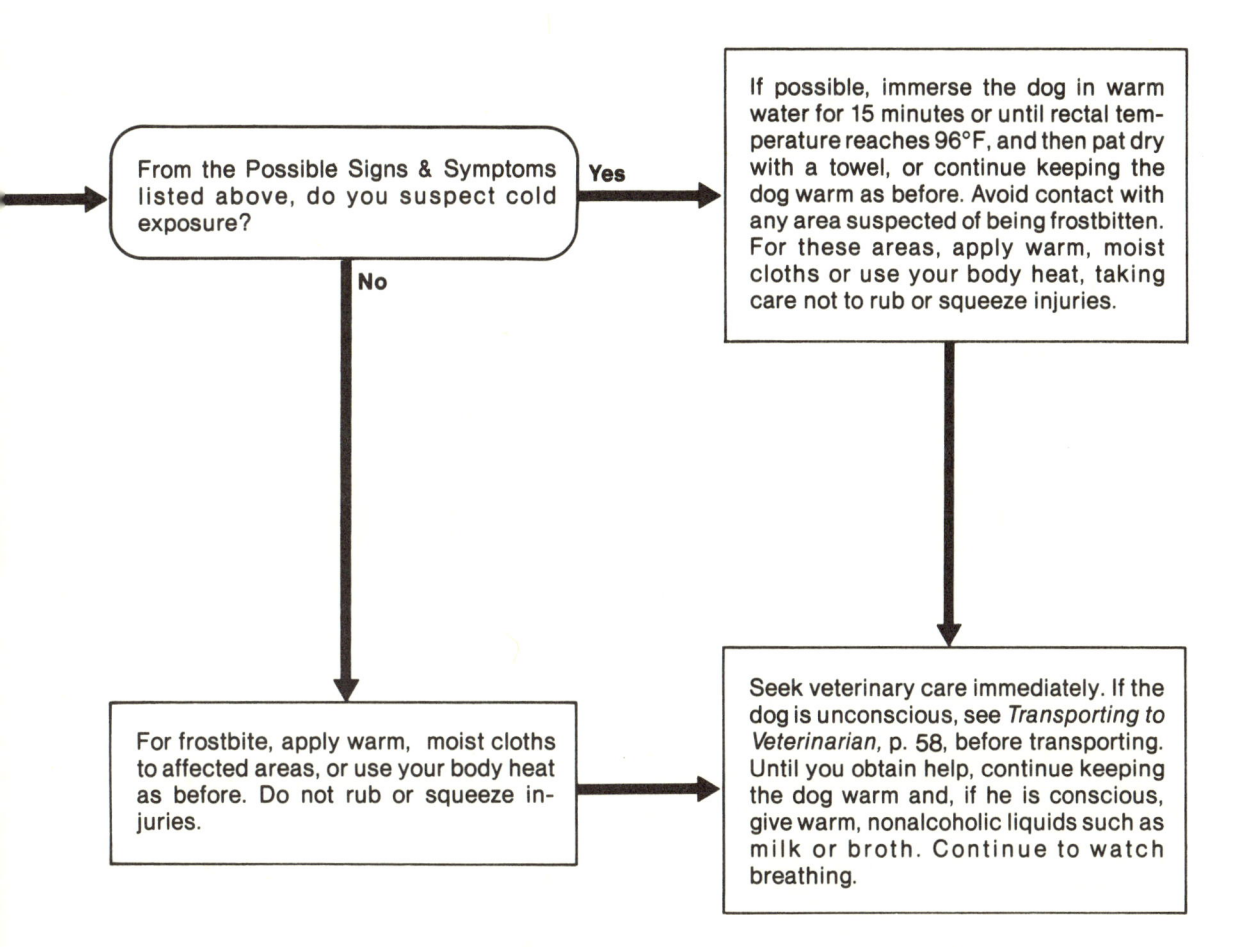

Calm the dog by speaking gently.

From the Possible Signs & Symptoms listed above, do you suspect cold exposure?

Yes → If possible, immerse the dog in warm water for 15 minutes or until rectal temperature reaches 96°F, and then pat dry with a towel, or continue keeping the dog warm as before. Avoid contact with any area suspected of being frostbitten. For these areas, apply warm, moist cloths or use your body heat, taking care not to rub or squeeze injuries.

No ↓

For frostbite, apply warm, moist cloths to affected areas, or use your body heat as before. Do not rub or squeeze injuries.

→ Seek veterinary care immediately. If the dog is unconscious, see *Transporting to Veterinarian,* p. 58, before transporting. Until you obtain help, continue keeping the dog warm and, if he is conscious, give warm, nonalcoholic liquids such as milk or broth. Continue to watch breathing.

---

*Do not muzzle, or if muzzled, remove immediately, if the dog is unconscious, convulsing, vomiting, having difficulty breathing, or there is blood or other matter in mouth.

Heatstroke & Heat Exhaustion

Never leave a dog in a hot, unventilated area (such as a car with closed windows) even for a few minutes.

→ Restrain the dog, if necessary. (See Restraining Procedure box.) If possible, bring the dog indoors to a cool room. Cool with an air conditioner or an electric fan, or open windows and fan the dog vigorously. Outdoors, move the dog to a shaded area.

Restraining Procedure:
*Muzzling:** For a short-nosed dog, wrap a thick towel firmly around head and neck, securing ends. For a long-nosed dog, bring a long gauze or cloth strip under chin; make a single half-knot on top, bring back under chin, tie a single half-knot again, and bring ends behind head, tying securely into a bow. Do not knot.
Move the dog if in an unsafe area.
Restraining: If the dog is not lying down, straddle his back, facing his head. Gently but firmly hold him with your legs. To have him sit, press on hind quarters; to have him lie, apply firm, gentle pressure gradually to upper back.
— If there are two persons, second person can now treat the dog.
— If you are alone, hold the dog firmly with your legs and one arm, or strap with ties, belts, etc., before treating.

Has breathing stopped?

Yes → See *Artificial Respiration & CPR*, p. 60. When breathing resumes, return to this chart.

No → Take the dog's temperature. (See p. 51.)

*Do not muzzle, or if muzzled, remove immediately, if the dog is unconscious, convulsing, vomiting, having difficulty breathing, or there is blood or other matter in mouth.

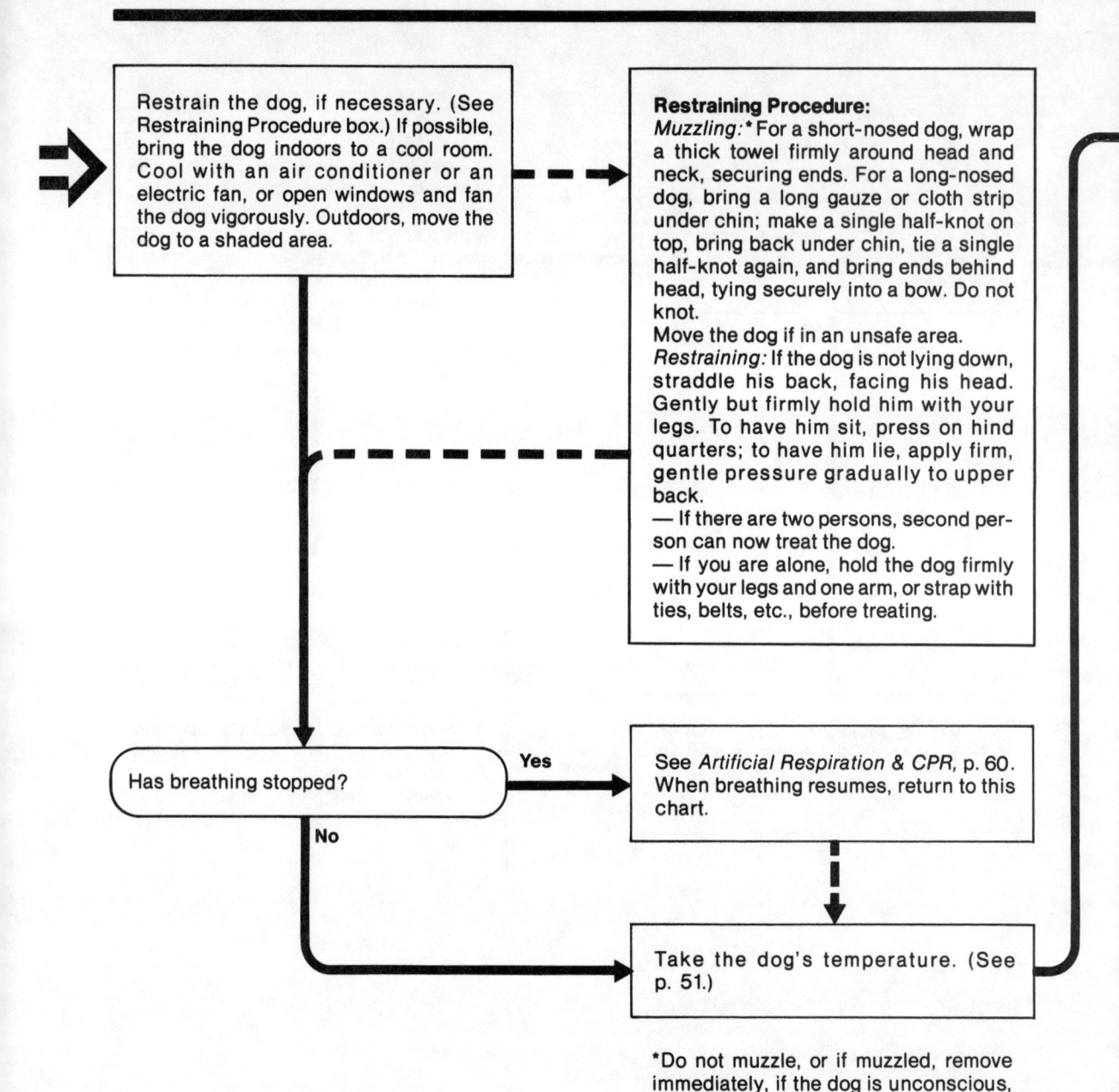

Possible Signs & Symptoms: *vomiting/diarrhea/panting or rapid breathing/foaming at the mouth/blue or grey tongue and gums/loss of consciousness. Heatstroke will be accompanied by a temperature of 106°F; heat exhaustion may not be accompanied by a fever.*

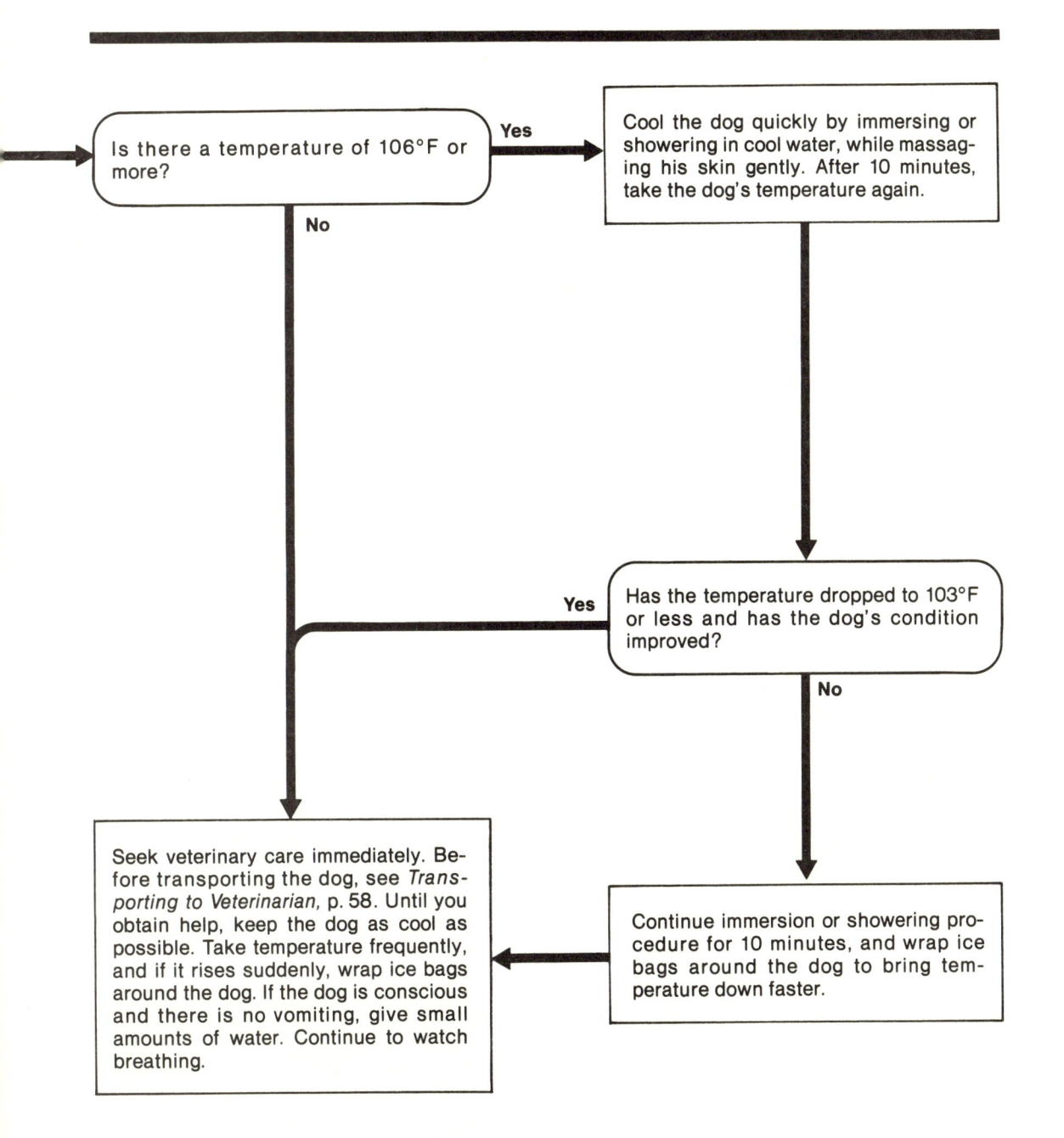

Calm the dog by speaking gently.

Is there a temperature of 106°F or more?

Yes → Cool the dog quickly by immersing or showering in cool water, while massaging his skin gently. After 10 minutes, take the dog's temperature again.

No ↓

Has the temperature dropped to 103°F or less and has the dog's condition improved?

Yes ←

No ↓

Continue immersion or showering procedure for 10 minutes, and wrap ice bags around the dog to bring temperature down faster.

Seek veterinary care immediately. Before transporting the dog, see *Transporting to Veterinarian,* p. 58. Until you obtain help, keep the dog as cool as possible. Take temperature frequently, and if it rises suddenly, wrap ice bags around the dog. If the dog is conscious and there is no vomiting, give small amounts of water. Continue to watch breathing.

Acknowledgements

While preparing *Your Dog: An Owner's Manual*, we sought advice from a number of experts in the veterinary, medical, and dog care fields. We are grateful to all those who graciously gave their time and expertise, including the consultants listed on page iii and Elihu B. Boroson, DVM; Steven Haskins, DVM; Henry J. Heimlich, MD; Ronald Kolata, DVM; Carol S. Moulton, Editor, *The Humane Society of the United States News*; Peter M. Schantz, VMD, The Center for Disease Control; and Ira Zaslow, DVM.

We would also like to express our appreciation to Tom Fowler, Denta Porter, and Bill Feeney of Tom Fowler, Inc., who literally worked day and night on the design and illustrations for this book.

And our special thanks to "Bear," who assisted Brian Kilcommons in demonstrating his training methods, and to "Ronnie," who patiently posed for the manual's canine illustrations.

NOTES

NOTES

NOTES

NOTES